T0296911

.

**Second Edition**

## CRAM SESSION IN

# Goniometry and Manual Muscle Testing

A Handbook for Students & Clinicians

**Second Edition**

# CRAM SESSION IN
# Goniometry and Manual Muscle Testing

A Handbook for Students & Clinicians

## Lynn Van Ost, MEd, RN, PT, ATC
Doctors of Physical Therapy, LLC
Plainfield, Illinois

## Jenna Morogiello, DAT, LAT, ATC, CSCS
United States Military Academy at West Point
West Point, New York

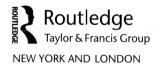
Routledge
Taylor & Francis Group
NEW YORK AND LONDON

First published 2023 by SLACK Incorporated

Published 2024 by Routledge
605 Third Avenue, New York, NY 10158

and by Routledge
4 Park Square, Milton Park, Abingdon, Oxon OX14 4RN

*Routledge is an imprint of the Taylor & Francis Group, an informa business*

Cover: Tinhouse Design

Library of Congress Cataloging-in-Publication Data

Names: Van Ost, Lynn, author. | Morogiello, Jenna, author.
Title: Cram session in goniometry and manual muscle testing : a handbook for students & clinicians / Lynn Van Ost, Jenna Morogiello.
Description: Second edition. | Thorofare, NJ : SLACK Incorporated, [2022] | Includes bibliographical references and index.
Identifiers: LCCN 2022030155 (print) | ISBN 9781630919894 (paperback) |
Subjects: MESH: Arthrometry, Articular--methods | Muscle Strength--physiology | Muscle Weakness--diagnosis | Handbook
Classification: LCC RD734 (print) | NLM WE 39 | DDC 616.7/40754--dc23/eng/20220810
LC record available at https://lccn.loc.gov/2022030155

ISBN: 9781630919894 (pbk)
ISBN: 9781003523413 (ebk)

DOI: 10.4324/9781003523413

# Dedication

To my dad, William C. Van Ost, MD, who always encouraged me to continue to grab for the next rung on the ladder.

*—Lynn Van Ost, MEd, RN, PT, ATC*

To my parents, Nancy and Dan Morogiello, whose unconditional love never ceases to inspire me.

*—Jenna Morogiello, DAT, LAT, ATC, CSCS*

# Contents

## GONIOMETRY

# Acknowledgments

We would like to thank the many individuals who assisted us in order to make this project possible. First and foremost, those at SLACK Incorporated: Tony Schiavo and the whole production team whose support has been endless. We are grateful for your professionalism and guidance.

We are indebted to Michael Raymond, Andrew Overman, Brian Lehrer, John Bear, and Cleveland Richard, who spent many hours being photographed for this manual. An additional thank you to Paige McHenry and Maddie Hansen for your flexibility and patience during our photo sessions. This book could not have been produced without your help. Our gratitude is also extended to Karen Manfré, Michelle Bartkowski, Jennifer Mintz, and Jenine LaFevere for many hours serving as the examiners in the photographs.

# About the Authors

*Lynn Van Ost, MEd, RN, PT, ATC,* graduated in 1982 with a bachelor's degree in nursing from West Chester State College in West Chester, Pennsylvania; was certified by the Board of Certification in athletic training in 1984; graduated in 1987 from Temple University in Philadelphia, Pennsylvania, with a master's degree in sports medicine/athletic training; and received a second bachelor's degree in physical therapy in 1988 from Temple University. In addition to treating the general orthopedic population as a physical therapist, she has worked with both amateur and professional athletes and has more than 11 years of experience as an athletic trainer working with Olympic-level elite athletes at numerous international events, including the 1992 and 1996 Summer Olympic games.

She currently works for Doctors of Physical Therapy, LLC as an Onsite Physical Therapist.

*Jenna Morogiello, DAT, LAT, ATC, CSCS,* graduated from West Chester University in 2015 with a bachelor's degree in athletic training and a minor in Spanish; Georgia Southern University in 2017 with a master's degree in kinesiology with a concentration in athletic training; and University of Idaho in 2020 with a clinical doctoral degree in athletic training. She was formerly the head athletic trainer for Campus Recreation and Intramurals at Georgia Southern University while serving as a preceptor and teacher in the master's of kinesiology program.

She currently serves as the Director of the Human Performance Lab, Assistant Professor of Kinesiology, and Certified Athletic Trainer in the Department of Physical Education for the United States Military Academy at West Point.

# Preface

There are many textbooks on the market dedicated either wholly or in part to the topics of goniometry and manual muscle testing; however, there are few books available that serve as a standalone quick reference for the clinician or student. The idea behind this manual was born from the need for a reference that would supply the clinician or student with a snapshot view of the basics of goniometry and manual muscle testing. This manual was not designed or intended as a teaching tool or as an introductory text on the subjects of goniometry or manual muscle testing. It does not contain information on the theories, validity, or reliability of goniometry or manual muscle testing; other textbooks cover those areas sufficiently. This book is intended to be a simple, user-friendly reference for the experienced clinician or student.

Although this manual was primarily intended for use by physical therapists, athletic trainers, and occupational therapists, its use is not limited to those specialties. It could easily find a home on the office shelf of any health care provider who performs musculoskeletal examinations.

This text is organized by body region in a "head-to-toe" format to make it easier and more efficient to locate a specific test. In the Goniometry section of this manual, each region is broken down into a description of type of joint, capsular pattern, average range of motion for each movement, patient positioning, goniometric alignment, alternative methods of measurement, and patient substitutions. The Manual Muscle Testing section of this manual is subdivided into the specific movement to be tested, active range of motion, the prime movers of the movement, the secondary movers, the anti-gravity patient position, gravity minimized patient position, stabilization and grades, substitutions for the movement, and points of interest for that particular muscle group. There are more than 200 photographs in the Goniometry section and more than 230 photographs in the Manual Muscle Testing section of this manual, illustrating the tests described. Although body part stabilization is described in the Goniometry section of the manual, it is not always pictured to allow for better visualization of joint movement in the photographs. Finally, there are 10 appendices listed in the back of this book. The first 5 appendices supplement the Goniometry section and describe procedure for measurement, goniometric terminology, average values of adult joint range of motion, anatomical zero, and capsular patterns. The next 4 appendices supplement the Manual Muscle Testing section and list manual muscle testing grading, general procedures for testing, manual muscle testing terminology, and factors that may cause inaccurate muscle testing and precautions/contraindications for manual muscle testing. The final appendix addresses sample and additional tools for goniometry/muscle strength testing if the examiner requires a more precise measurement. The authors took care to present this manual in a clear, concise manner. If it makes the tasks of taking goniometric measurements and performing manual muscle tests easier and more accurate for the clinician, then the goal of this manual will have been achieved.

# GONIOMETRY

# SECTION I

# Cervical Spine

# THE CERVICAL SPINE

**Type of joint:** The cervical spine is made up of a series of joints allowing for 3 degrees of freedom of the neck. The goniometer is only capable of measuring gross movements of the cervical spine; individual types of joints (eg, the atlantoccipital or atlantoaxial joints) will not be addressed in this section.

**Capsular pattern:** Lateral flexion = rotation/extension.

## Cervical Flexion

**Planes/axis of movement:** Movement occurs in the sagittal plane around a coronal axis. It includes all segmental movements of the occiput, cervical, and thoracic vertebrae to approximately T7.

**Range of motion:**

- 0 degrees to 45 degrees with the goniometer

- 1.0 cm to 4.3 cm with tape measure

**Preferred starting position:** See Figure 1-1.

**End position:** See Figure 1-2.

**Goniometric alignment:**

- Axis: Center over the external auditory meatus

- Stationary arm: Align perpendicular to the floor

- Moving arm: Align parallel to the base of the nose

**Stabilization:** The trunk should be stabilized against the back of a chair.

**Substitutions:** The examiner must watch to make sure the patient does not flex the trunk or laterally bend/rotate the head during testing. These substitutions are commonly seen if the tested motion causes pain.

**Alternate method/position for testing:** See Figure 1-3.

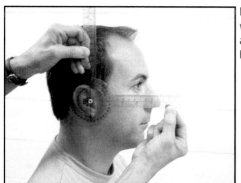

**Figure 1-1**. The patient should be sitting with the thoracic spine stabilized against a chair. The head is in neutral position. The hands should be in the patient's lap.

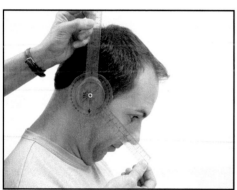

**Figure 1-2**. The cervical spine should be in a position of maximal flexion at the end of the movement.

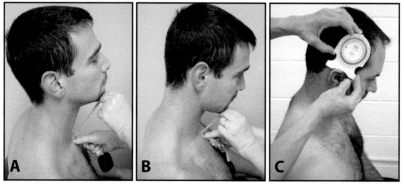

**Figure 1-3**. A tape measure may be used in place of a goniometer. The distance is measured between the chin and sternal notch. The patient's mouth should be closed during testing. (A) Alternate starting position. (B) End position. (C) A fluid goniometer may also be used with the base resting on top of the ear.

GONIO

# Cervical Extension/Hyperextension

**Planes/axis of movement:** Movement occurs in the sagittal plane around a coronal axis. It includes all segmental movements of the occiput, cervical, and thoracic vertebrae to approximately T7. Movement beyond neutral is considered hyperextension.

**Range of motion:**

· 45 degrees to 0 degrees of extension (from full flexion)

· 0 degrees to 45 degrees of hyperextension

· Approximately 7 inches of extension, using a tape measure

· Approximately 10 inches of hyperextension (from full flexion) using a tape measure

**Preferred starting position:** See Figure 1-4.

**End position:** See Figure 1-5.

**Goniometric alignment:**

· Axis: Center over the external auditory meatus

· Stationary arm: Align perpendicular to the floor

· Moving arm: Align parallel to the base of the nose

**Stabilization:** The trunk should be stabilized against the back of a chair.

**Substitutions:** The patient may try to extend the trunk or laterally bend/rotate the head during testing. These substitutions are commonly seen if the tested motion causes pain.

**Alternate method/position for testing:** See Figure 1-6.

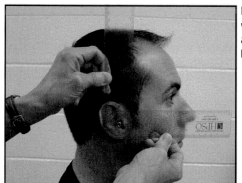

**Figure 1-4**. The patient should be sitting with the thoracic spine stabilized against a chair. The head is in neutral position. The hands should be in the patient's lap.

GONIO

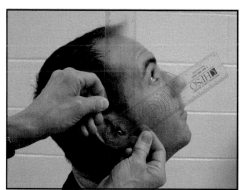

**Figure 1-5**. The cervical spine should be in full cervical extension/hyperextension at the end of the movement.

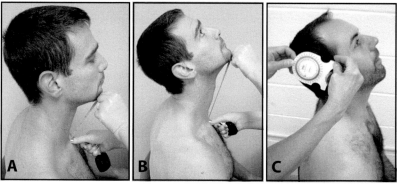

**Figure 1-6**. A tape measure may be used in place of a goniometer. The distance is measured between the chin and the sternal notch. (A) Alternate starting position. (B) End position. (C) A fluid goniometer may also be used with the base resting on top of the ear.

GONIO

# Cervical Lateral Flexion

**Planes/axis of movement:** Movement occurs in the frontal plane around an anterior/posterior axis and occurs segmentally along the cervical vertebrae. There is a component of rotation that occurs to allow for full movement of the head.

**Range of motion:**

- 0 degrees to 45 degrees

- Approximately 5 inches if using a tape measure

**Preferred starting position:** See Figure 1-7.

**End position:** See Figure 1-8.

**Goniometric alignment:**

- Axis: Center over the spinous process of C7

- Stationary arm: Align perpendicular to the floor

- Moving arm: Align over the external occipital protuberance of the occiput

**Stabilization:** The trunk should be stabilized against the back of a chair. Additional stabilization is achieved by holding the patient's shoulder down with the clinician's hand.

**Substitutions:** The patient may try to laterally flex the trunk or rotate the head to increase the range of motion or avoid pain with movement.

**Alternate method/position for testing:** See Figure 1-9.

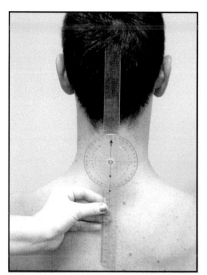
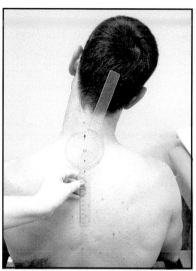

**Figure 1-7**. The patient should be sitting with the thoracic spine stabilized against a chair. The head is in a neutral position. The hands should be in the patient's lap.

**Figure 1-8**. The cervical spine should be in full lateral cervical flexion at the end of the movement.

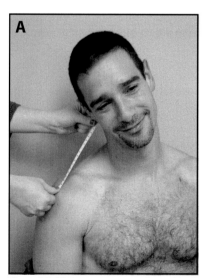
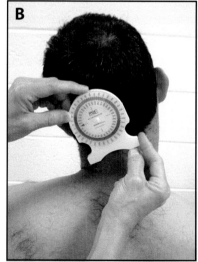

**Figure 1-9**. (A) A tape measure may be used in place of a goniometer. The distance between the mastoid process and acromion process is measured. It is important to measure and record the differences in length between the starting position and end position in determining the range of motion. (B) A fluid goniometer may also be used with the base aligned with the external occipital protuberance.

## Cervical Rotation

**Planes/axis of movement:** Movement occurs in the transverse plane around a vertical axis. Most of this motion occurs at the atlantoaxial joint (C1-C2). Some cervical lateral flexion to the same side of the rotation should occur during movement.

**Range of motion:**

- 0 degrees to 60 degrees
- Approximately 5 inches if using a tape measure

**Preferred starting position:** See Figure 1-10.

**End position:** See Figure 1-11.

**Goniometric alignment:**

- Axis: Align over the center of the top of the head
- Stationary arm: Align with the acromion process of the tested side
- Moving arm: Align with the tip of the nose

**Stabilization:** The trunk should be stabilized against the back of a chair.

**Substitutions:** The patient may try to rotate the trunk, laterally flex the neck, or elevate the scapula to the tested side to avoid pain during the movement.

**Alternate method/position for testing:** See Figure 1-12.

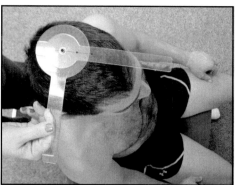

**Figure 1-10**. The patient should be sitting with the head in neutral position and the hands in the patient's lap.

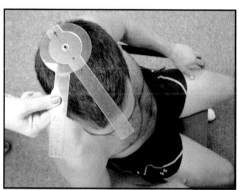

**Figure 1-11**. The cervical spine should be in full cervical rotation at the end of the movement.

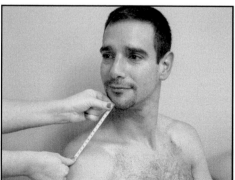

**Figure 1-12**. A tape measure may be used in place of a goniometer. The distance between the top of the chin and the same side acromion process is measured. It is important to measure and record the differences in length between the starting position and end position in determining the range of motion.

GONIO

# THE SCAPULOTHORACIC JOINT

**Type of joint:** Movements relating to the scapula sliding over the thorax are described as movements of the scapulothoracic joint. This is a "functional" joint in which there are no typical joint characteristics. All movements of the scapula and scapulothoracic joint are intimately related to the sternoclavicular and acromioclavicular joints, but these joint articulations will not be discussed as they cannot be measured with a goniometer. The best method for determining scapulothoracic joint movement is by the use of a tape measure.

**Capsular pattern:** None.

## Scapular Upward Rotation

**Planes/axis of movement:** Motion occurs in the frontal plane around an anterior/posterior axis during glenohumeral abduction and flexion. The inferior angle of the scapula moves away from the vertebral column.

**Range of motion:**

- Normal range of motion is determined by comparing the motion of one scapula to the other. The measurement is recorded in inches or centimeters between the anatomical starting and ending positions.

**Preferred starting position:** See Figure 2-1.

**End position:** See Figure 2-2.

**Goniometric alignment points:** The inferior angle of the scapula and the spinous process of the seventh thoracic vertebra T7 are palpated and identified.

**Measurement of motion:** The distance between the inferior angle of the scapula and the spinous process of the seventh thoracic vertebra T7 is measured. The patient fully abducts the shoulder and a second measurement is taken. The difference between the 2 measurements is the amount of scapular upward rotation present.

**Stabilization:** Thoracic stabilization is achieved through patient compliance.

**Substitutions:** The patient may attempt to laterally flex or extend the trunk to gain more shoulder motion. This may be more commonly seen in individuals with upper extremity weakness or those with glenohumeral limitations.

**Alternate method/position for testing:** See Figure 2-3.

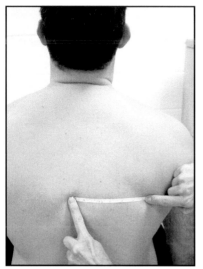

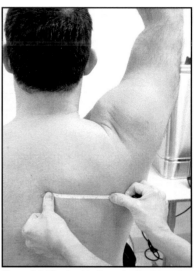

**Figure 2-1**. The patient should sit with the shoulder in anatomical position. The upper extremity should be in a neutral position.

**Figure 2-2**. The shoulder is maximally abducted or flexed to allow for full scapular upward rotation.

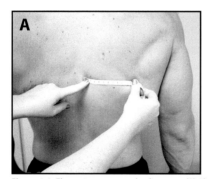

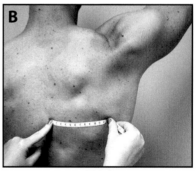

**Figure 2-3**. The patient may stand or lie prone. (A) Alternate starting position. (B) End position.

# Scapular Downward Rotation

**Planes/axis of movement:** Motion occurs in the frontal plane around an anterior/posterior axis. Downward rotation of the scapula is a rotary movement of the inferior angle toward the vertebral column. It occurs during shoulder adduction and extension across the posterior trunk.

**Range of motion:**

- Normal range of motion is determined by comparing the motion of one scapula to the other. The measurement is recorded in inches or centimeters between the anatomical starting position and ending position.

**Preferred starting position:** See Figure 2-4.

**End position:** See Figure 2-5.

**Goniometric alignment points:** The inferior angle of the scapula and the spinous process of the T7 vertebra are palpated and identified.

**Measurement of motion:** The distance between the inferior angle of the scapula and the spinous process of T7 is measured. The patient fully adducts the upper limb across the posterior trunk and a second measurement is taken. The difference between the 2 measurements is the amount of scapular downward rotation present.

**Stabilization:** Thoracic stabilization is achieved through patient compliance.

**Substitutions:** The patient may try to retract the scapula to gain more motion. This may be seen in individuals with range of motion limitations at the glenohumeral joint.

**Alternate method/position for testing:** See Figure 2-6.

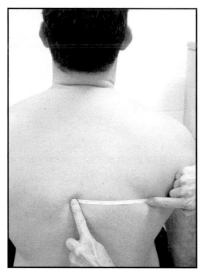 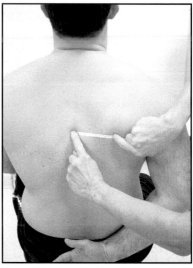

**Figure 2-4**. The patient should sit with the shoulder in anatomical position. The upper extremity should be in a neutral position.

**Figure 2-5**. The patient is asked to maximally extend and adduct their arm across their back.

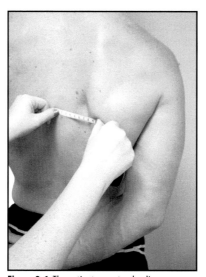

**Figure 2-6**. The patient may stand or lie prone.

# Scapular Abduction

**Planes/axis of movement:** Motion occurs in the frontal plane and is translatory. The scapula moves laterally across the thorax as the shoulder is horizontally adducted in the transverse plane.

**Preferred starting position:** See Figure 2-7.

**End position:** See Figure 2-8.

**Goniometric alignment points:** The origin or root of the spine of the scapula is palpated and identified. The corresponding thoracic vertebra at that level is also palpated and identified.

**Measurement of motion:** The distance between the origin of the spine of the scapula and the thoracic vertebrae is measured. The patient fully horizontally adducts the shoulder across the anterior trunk and a second measurement is taken. The difference between the 2 measurements is the amount of scapular abduction present.

**Stabilization:** Thoracic stabilization is achieved through patient compliance.

**Substitutions:** The examiner must be aware of the individual trying to rotate the glenohumeral joint or laterally flex the trunk to gain more motion or avoid pain during the motion.

**Alternate method/position for testing:** None.

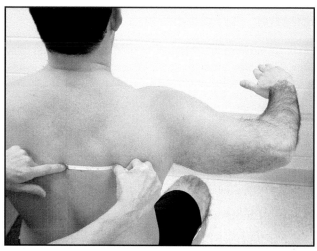

**Figure 2-7**. The patient should be sitting with the shoulder in 90 degrees of abduction. The elbow should be flexed to 90 degrees; the forearm and wrist should be in neutral positions.

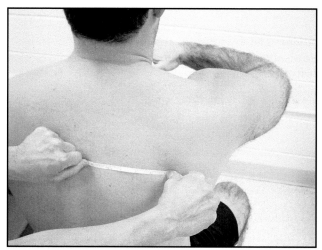

**Figure 2-8**. The patient is asked to horizontally adduct their arm maximally across their chest.

# Scapular Adduction

**Planes/axis of movement:** Motion occurs in the frontal plane and is translatory. The scapula moves medially across the thorax as the shoulder is horizontally abducted in the transverse plane.

**Preferred starting position:** See Figure 2-9.

**End position:** See Figure 2-10.

**Goniometric alignment points:** The origin or root of the spine of the scapula is palpated and identified. The corresponding thoracic vertebra at that level is also palpated and marked.

**Measurement of motion:** The distance between the origin of the spine of the scapula and the thoracic vertebrae is measured. The patient fully horizontally abducts the shoulder across the posterior trunk and a second measurement is taken. The difference between the 2 measurements is the amount of scapular adduction present.

**Stabilization:** Thoracic stabilization is achieved through patient compliance.

**Substitutions:** The examiner must be aware of the individual trying to rotate the shoulder joint or rotate the trunk to gain more motion or avoid pain during the movement.

**Alternate method/position for testing:** None.

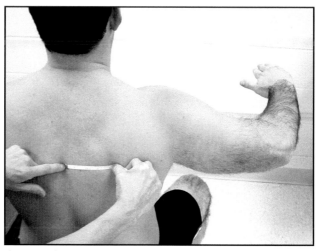

**Figure 2-9.** The patient should be sitting with the shoulder in 90 degrees of abduction. The elbow should be flexed to 90 degrees; the forearm and wrist should be in neutral positions.

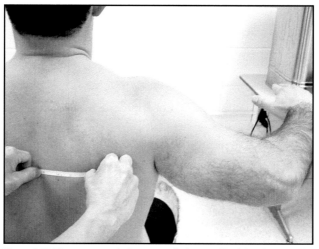

**Figure 2-10.** The patient is asked to maximally horizontally abduct their shoulder across the posterior thorax.

# THE SHOULDER (GLENOHUMERAL JOINT)

**Type of joint:** Ball and socket joint with 3 degrees of freedom allowing for flexion/extension, abduction/adduction, and internal/external rotation. The anatomic axis is through the center of the head of the humerus.

**Capsular pattern:** External rotation > abduction > internal rotation.

## Shoulder Flexion

**Planes/axis of movement:** Motion occurs in the sagittal plane around a transverse axis through the head of the humerus.

**Range of motion:**

- 0 degrees to 180 degrees

**Preferred starting position:** See Figure 2-11.

**End position:** See Figure 2-12.

**Goniometric alignment:**

- Axis: Near the acromion process, through the humeral head

- Stationary arm: Align with the midaxillary line of the trunk

- Moving arm: Align with the lateral midline of the humerus siting the lateral epicondyle of the humerus

**Stabilization:** The scapula must be stabilized against a supporting surface by the weight of the trunk to prevent elevation, upward rotation, and posterior tilting. The clinician may use their hand to stabilize the scapula if the patient is in sitting.

**Substitutions:** Common substitutions in an attempt to gain more shoulder flexion may include lumbar hyperextension, shoulder abduction, or scapular elevation. These substitutions may occur because of limitations at the glenohumeral joint or as a result of pain during testing.

**Alternate method/position for testing:** See Figures 2-13A and 2-13B.

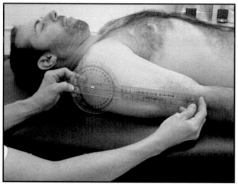

**Figure 2-11.** The patient is positioned in supine with the knees flexed to stabilize the lumbar spine. The elbow is extended and the forearm is in midposition between supination and pronation.

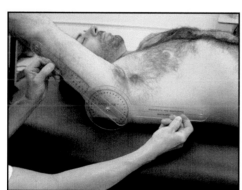

**Figure 2-12.** The shoulder should be in a position of maximal flexion at the end of the movement. The elbow should be in extension, and the forearm should be in a neutral position.

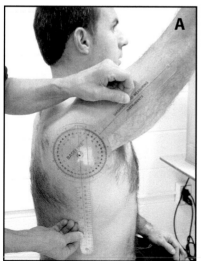
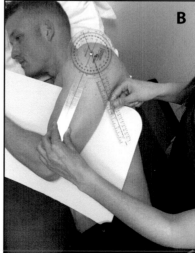

**Figure 2-13.** The patient may be placed in sitting (A) or sidelying with slide board underneath the shoulder (B).

GONIO

GONIO

# Shoulder Extension/ Hyperextension

**Planes/axis of movement:** Motion occurs in the sagittal plane around a transverse axis through the head of the humerus. Extension is the reverse action of flexion. As the arm passes the trunk in the anatomic position, hyperextension occurs.

**Range of motion:**

- 180 degrees to 0 degrees of extension (from full flexion)

- 0 degrees to 40 to 60 degrees of hyperextension

**Preferred starting position:** See Figure 2-14.

**End position:** See Figure 2-15.

**Goniometric alignment:**

- Axis: Near the acromion process, through the humeral head

- Stationary arm: Align with the midaxillary line of the trunk

- Moving arm: Align with the lateral midline of the humerus siting the lateral epicondyle of the humerus

**Stabilization:** The scapula should be stabilized against a supporting surface by the weight of the trunk to prevent anterior tilting and elevation. The clinician may use their hand to stabilize the scapula if the patient is in sitting.

**Substitutions:** The patient may try to extend the trunk or abduct the shoulder to complete the motion or avoid pain during testing.

**Alternate method/position for testing:** See Figure 2-16.

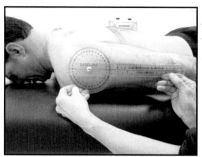

**Figure 2-14**. The patient is placed in the prone position with the forearm in midposition between supination and pronation. The head should not be supported by a pillow, and the elbow should be slightly flexed.

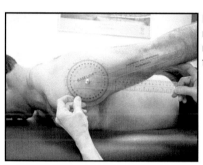

**Figure 2-15**. The shoulder should be in a position of maximal extension/hyperextension at the end of the movement. The elbow should be in extension with the forearm in a pronated position.

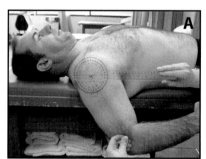

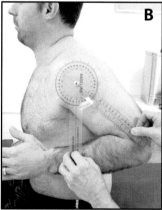

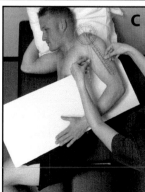

**Figure 2-16**. The patient may be placed in the supine position (A) with the arm resting over the side of the table, in sitting (B), or in sidelying with a slide board (C).

# Shoulder Abduction

**Planes/axis of movement:** Motion occurs in the frontal plane around an anterior/posterior axis.

**Range of motion:**

- 0 degrees to 180 degrees

**Preferred starting position:** See Figure 2-17.

**End position:** See Figure 2-18.

**Goniometric alignment:**

- Axis: Close to the anterior aspect of the acromion process through the center of the humeral head

- Stationary arm: Align parallel to the midline of the sternum along the lateral aspect of the trunk

- Moving arm: Align along the medial midline of the humerus siting the medial epicondyle of the humerus

**Stabilization:** The scapula must be stabilized against a supporting surface by the weight of the trunk. The clinician may also use their hand to stabilize the clavicle and scapula if necessary to prevent elevation and upward rotation.

**Substitutions:** The examiner should not allow the patient to elevate the scapula or laterally flex the trunk to the contralateral side during testing in an attempt to gain more range of motion. Allow the shoulder to externally rotate during testing.

**Alternate method/position for testing:** See Figure 2-19.

**Goniometric alignment if testing in sitting:**

- Axis: Posterior aspect of the acromion process, through the center of the humeral head

- Stationary arm: Align parallel to the spinous process of the vertebral column

- Moving arm: Align on the posterior aspect of the humeral shaft, siting the olecranon process of the ulna

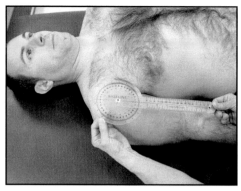

**Figure 2-17**. The patient should be placed in the supine position. The shoulder should be in midposition between flexion and extension with the shoulder in full external rotation. The forearm should be in midposition between supination and pronation with the elbow in full extension.

GONIO

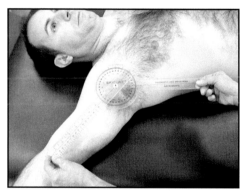

**Figure 2-18**. The shoulder should be in a position of maximal abduction at the end of the movement.

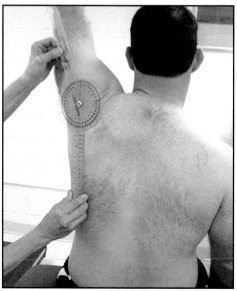

**Figure 2-19**. The patient may be placed in a prone or sitting position.

# Shoulder Adduction

**Planes/axis of movement:** Movement occurs in the frontal plane around an anterior/posterior axis. It is discontinued by contact of the upper arm with the body.

**Range of motion:**

- 180 degrees to 0 degrees (from full abduction)

**Preferred starting position:** See Figure 2-20.

**End position:** See Figure 2-21.

**Goniometric alignment:**

- Axis: Anterior aspect of the acromion process, through the center of the humeral head

- Stationary arm: Align along the lateral aspect of the anterior surface of the trunk in parallel with the midline of the sternum

- Moving arm: Align with the midline of the humerus siting the medial epicondyle of the humerus

**Stabilization:** Stabilize the thorax against a supporting surface and encourage patient compliance to prevent ipsilateral flexion. Allow the shoulder to internally rotate.

**Substitutions:** The patient may try to laterally flex the trunk toward the tested side to gain more motion or avoid pain during testing.

**Alternate method/position for testing:** The patient may be placed in a sitting position.

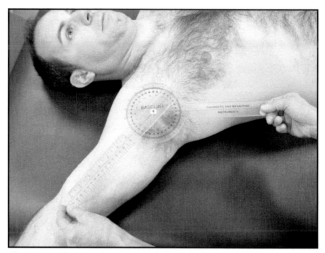

**Figure 2-20**. The patient lies supine with the shoulder in a maximally abducted and externally rotated position.

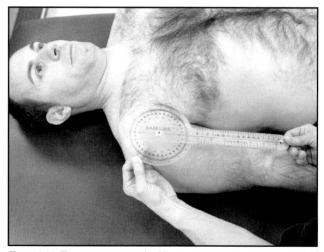

**Figure 2-21**. The upper extremity should come to rest at the maximum range of shoulder adduction.

# Shoulder Horizontal Abduction

**Planes/axis of movement:** Movement occurs in the transverse plane around a vertical axis. The scapula adducts on the thorax during movement.

**Range of motion:**

- 0 degrees to 45 degrees from neutral
- 0 degrees to 135 degrees from a fully horizontally adducted position

**Preferred starting position:** See Figure 2-22.

**End position:** See Figure 2-23.

**Goniometric alignment:**

- Axis: The superior aspect of the acromion process through the head of the humerus
- Stationary arm: Align along the midline of the shoulder siting the base of the neck
- Moving arm: Align along the midline of the humeral shaft, siting the lateral epicondyle of the humerus

**Stabilization:** The thorax must be stabilized against the back of a chair to prevent trunk rotation.

**Substitutions:** The patient may attempt to rotate the trunk or laterally flex to the opposite side to gain more movement. Scapular elevation is also another substitution seen during testing.

**Alternate method/position for testing:** None.

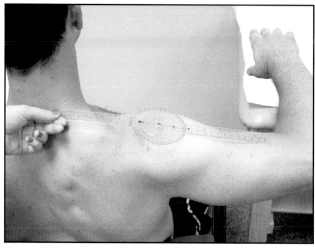

**Figure 2-22**. The patient should be sitting with the shoulder in neutral rotation. The shoulder should be abducted to 90 degrees with the elbow in 90 degrees of flexion.

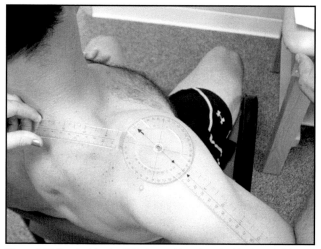

**Figure 2-23**. The shoulder should be in a position of maximal horizontal abduction with the scapula fully adducted.

# Shoulder Horizontal Adduction

**Planes/axis of movement:** Movement occurs in the transverse plane around a vertical axis. The scapula abducts on the thorax during the movement.

**Range of motion:**

- 0 degrees to 90 degrees from neutral
- 0 degrees to 135 degrees from a fully horizontally abducted position

**Preferred starting position:** See Figure 2-24.

**End position:** See Figure 2-25.

**Goniometric alignment:**

- Axis: The superior aspect of the acromion process of the scapula, through the head of the humerus
- Stationary arm: Align along the midline of the shoulder siting the base of the neck
- Moving arm: Align along the midline of the humeral shaft, siting the lateral epicondyle of the humerus

**Stabilization:** The thorax must be stabilized against the back of a chair or supporting surface to prevent rotation.

**Substitutions:** The patient may try to rotate the trunk to obtain more motion during testing.

**Alternate method/position for testing:** See Figure 2-26.

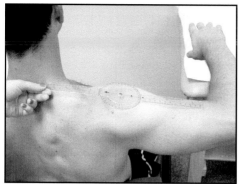

**Figure 2-24**. The patient should be sitting with the shoulder in neutral rotation. The shoulder joint is flexed to 90 degrees and the elbow is flexed to 90 degrees.

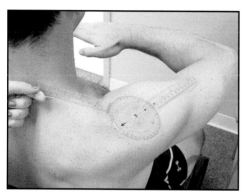

**Figure 2-25**. The shoulder should be in a position of maximal horizontal adduction at the end of the movement.

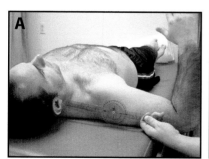

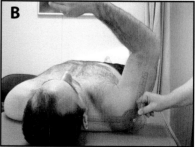

**Figure 2-26**. The patient lies in supine with the shoulder joint in 90 degrees abduction and neutral rotation and with the elbow in 90 degrees of flexion. (A) Alternate starting position. (B) End position.

GONIO

# Shoulder Internal (Medial) Rotation

**Planes/axis of movement:** Movement occurs in the transverse plane around a longitudinal axis through the head and shaft of the humerus.

**Range of motion:**

- With the shoulder stabilized: 0 degrees to 75 degrees
- Universally accepted range of motion: 0 degrees to 90 degrees

**Preferred starting position:** See Figure 2-27.

**End position:** See Figure 2-28.

**Goniometric alignment:**

- Axis: Over the olecranon process of the ulna
- Stationary arm: Align perpendicular to the floor
- Moving arm: Align with the shaft of the ulna, siting the styloid process of the ulna

**Stabilization:** Make sure the distal end of the humeral shaft is stabilized against a supporting surface and the trunk does not rise during the movement.

**Substitutions:** The trunk or anterior shoulder may elevate to accommodate a restricted joint capsule. The patient may also adduct or extend either the shoulder or elbow to avoid internally rotating the shoulder.

**Alternate method/position for testing:** See Figure 2-29.

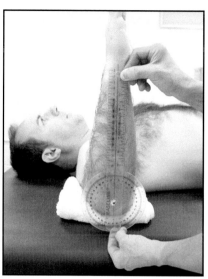

**Figure 2-27.** The patient should be in supine, with the shoulder joint positioned in 90 degrees of abduction. The forearm is placed in midposition between supination and pronation. The palm faces down toward the floor. The humerus is placed level with the acromion process by placing a pad under the upper arm. The elbow rests off the table.

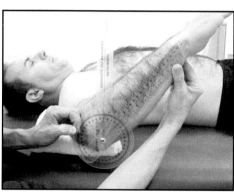

**Figure 2-28.** The shoulder should be in maximal internal rotation at the end of the movement with the palm facing the floor.

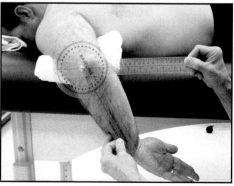

**Figure 2-29.** The patient may be placed in the prone position with the shoulder in 90 degrees abduction and with the elbow flexed to 90 degrees over the edge of the table.

**GONIO**

# Shoulder External (Lateral) Rotation

**Planes/axis of movement:** Motion occurs in the transverse plane around a longitudinal axis through the head and shaft of the humerus.

**Range of motion:**

- 0 degrees to 90 degrees

**Preferred starting position:** See Figure 2-30.

**End position:** See Figure 2-31.

**Goniometric alignment:**

- Axis: Over the olecranon process of the ulna

- Stationary arm: Align perpendicular to the floor

- Moving arm: Align with the shaft of the ulna, siting the styloid process of the ulna

**Stabilization:** Make sure the distal end of the humerus is stabilized against a supporting surface and the trunk does not rise during movement.

**Substitutions:** The examiner should watch carefully to make sure the patient does not extend the trunk or move the shoulder out of 90 degrees of abduction to avoid the movement. Elbow flexion or extension is another commonly seen substitution to avoid shoulder external rotation.

**Alternate method/position for testing:** The patient is in the prone position with the shoulder abducted to 90 degrees and the elbow flexed to 90 degrees over the edge of the table.

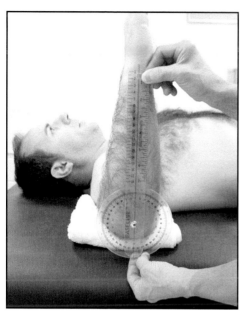

**Figure 2-30**. The patient should be lying in supine with the shoulder positioned in 90 degrees of abduction. The forearm is placed in midposition between supination and pronation. The palm faces down toward the floor. The humerus is placed level with the acromion process by placing a pad under the upper arm. The elbow rests off the table.

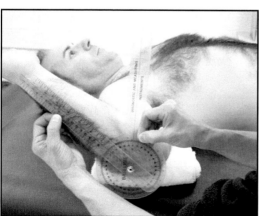

**Figure 2-31**. The shoulder should be in a position of maximal external rotation at the end of the movement.

GONIO

# THE ELBOW (HUMEROULNAR AND HUMERORADIAL JOINTS)

**Type of joint:** Hinge joint (ginglymus) with one degree of freedom allowing for flexion and extension.

**Capsular pattern:** Flexion > extension.

## Elbow Flexion

**Planes/axis of movement:** Motion occurs in the sagittal plane around a coronal axis.

**Range of motion:**

- 0 degrees to 145 degrees

**Preferred starting position:** See Figure 2-32.

**End position:** See Figure 2-33.

**Goniometric alignment:**

- Axis: Over the lateral epicondyle of the humerus
- Stationary arm: Align along the lateral midline of the humerus, siting the acromion process
- Moving arm: Align along the lateral midline of the radius, siting the radial styloid

**Stabilization:** The distal end of the humerus should be stabilized against a supporting surface to prevent shoulder flexion.

**Substitutions:** See Figure 2-34.

**Alternate method/position for testing:** See Figure 2-35.

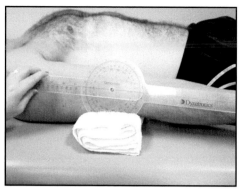

**Figure 2-32.** The patient lies supine with the upper arm close to the body. The shoulder should be in neutral position between flexion and extension. The forearm should be in supination. A pad should be placed at the distal end of the humerus to allow for full motion.

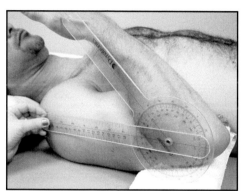

**Figure 2-33.** The elbow should be in maximal flexion at the end of the movement.

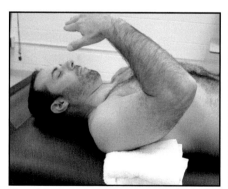

**Figure 2-34.** The patient may attempt to flex the shoulder to avoid pain or pronate the forearm to gain more motion during testing.

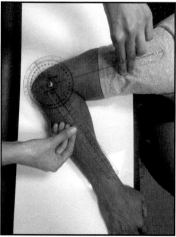

**Figure 2-35.** The patient may be placed in sitting with the forearm resting on a table top in a neutral position between pronation and supination.

# Elbow Extension

**Planes/axis of movement:** Movement occurs in the sagittal plane around a coronal axis.

**Range of motion:**

- 145 degrees to 0 degrees

**Preferred starting position:** See Figure 2-36.

**End position:** See Figure 2-37.

**Goniometric alignment:**

- Axis: On the lateral epicondyle of the humerus
- Stationary arm: Align along the lateral midline of the humerus, siting the acromion process
- Moving arm: Align along the lateral midline of the radius, siting the radial styloid

**Stabilization:** The proximal humerus should be stabilized anteriorly by the clinician's hand to prevent scapular protraction and trunk extension.

**Substitutions:** The patient may try to extend the trunk to enhance the motion or move the shoulder into flexion or extension to avoid pain with testing.

**Alternate method/position for testing:** None.

GONIO

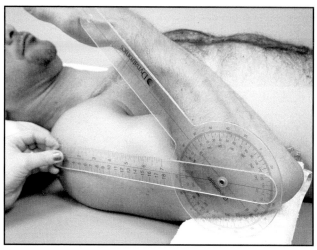

**Figure 2-36**. The patient is placed in a supine position with the upper arm alongside the trunk with the forearm in full supination and with the elbow maximally flexed.

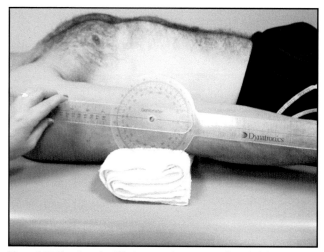

**Figure 2-37**. The elbow should be in maximal extension at the end of the movement.

# THE FOREARM (RADIOULNAR JOINT)

**Type of joint:** The proximal radioulnar joint may be considered alone as a uniaxial pivot joint with 1 degree of freedom.

**Capsular pattern:** Pronation = supination.

## Forearm Pronation

**Planes/axis of movement:** Motion occurs in the transverse plane around a longitudinal axis in the anatomical position. Motion occurs in the frontal plane while in the preferred testing position.

**Range of motion:**

- 0 degrees to 90 degrees

**Preferred starting position:** See Figure 2-38.

**End position:** See Figure 2-39.

**Goniometric alignment:**

- Axis: Lateral to the ulnar styloid

- Stationary arm: Align parallel to the anterior midline of the humerus

- Moving arm: Align across the dorsal aspect of the wrist, proximal to the styloid process of the ulna and radius

**Stabilization:** The distal end of the humerus must be stabilized on a supporting surface to prevent internal rotation and abduction at the shoulder joint. The patient may use the nontested hand to keep the humeral shaft against the thorax.

**Substitutions:** The patient may try to laterally flex the trunk away from the tested side or abduct/internally rotate the shoulder to increase the amount of range of motion.

**Alternate method/position for testing:** See Figure 2-40.

**Goniometric alignment for alternate method:**

- Axis: The third metacarpal head, siting through the third metacarpal shaft

- Stationary arm: Align perpendicular to the table surface

- Moving arm: Align parallel to the midline of the pencil

GONIO

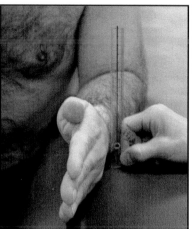

**Figure 2-38.** The patient is sitting with the shoulder in 0 degrees of abduction, flexion, and extension and with the elbow flexed to 90 degrees. The forearm should be in midposition between pronation and supination resting on a table top.

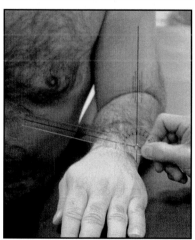

**Figure 2-39.** The forearm should be in a position of maximal pronation at the end of the movement.

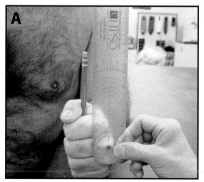
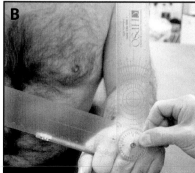

**Figure 2-40.** The patient may be in sitting gripping a pencil or pen vertically in their hand. (A) Alternate starting position. (B) End position.

# Forearm Supination

**Planes/axis of movement:** Movement occurs in the transverse plane around a longitudinal axis in the anatomical position. Motion occurs in the frontal plane while in the preferred testing position.

**Range of motion:**

- 0 degrees to 90 degrees

**Preferred starting position:** See Figure 2-41.

**End position:** See Figure 2-42.

**Goniometric alignment:**

- Axis: Center medial to the ulnar styloid process

- Stationary arm: Align on the anterior surface of the wrist parallel to the anterior midline of the humerus

- Moving arm: Place on the ventral surface of the wrist, just proximal to the styloid process of the ulna and radius

**Stabilization:** The humerus must be stabilized on a supporting surface to prevent external rotation of the shoulder. The patient may use the nontested hand to keep the humeral shaft against the thorax.

**Substitutions:** The patient may try to use shoulder external rotation to avoid a painful motion. The examiner may also observe the patient laterally flexing to the tested side or extending the elbow to obtain more movement.

**Alternate method/position for testing:** See Figure 2-43.

**Goniometric alignment for alternate method:**

- Axis: The third metacarpal head, siting through the third metacarpal shaft

- Stationary arm: Align perpendicular to the table surface

- Moving arm: Align parallel to the midline of the pencil

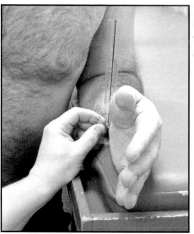

**Figure 2-41**. The patient is sitting with the shoulder in 0 degrees abduction, flexion, and extension. The forearm is placed in midposition between supination and pronation, resting on a table top.

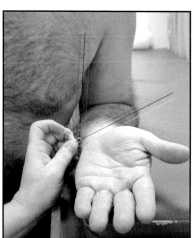

**Figure 2-42**. The forearm should be in a position of maximal supination at the end of the motion.

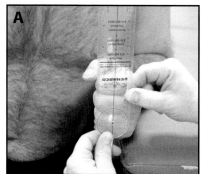
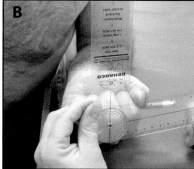

**Figure 2-43**. The patient may be in a sitting position gripping a pencil or pen vertically in their hand. (A) Alternate starting position. (B) End position.

# THE WRIST (RADIOCARPAL AND INTERCARPAL JOINTS)

**Type of joint:** This joint is classified as a condyloid joint with 2 degrees of freedom (flexion and extension, radial and ulnar deviation). The articulation of the proximal and distal rows of metacarpals are of the same classification and also allow for flexion and extension.

**Capsular pattern:** Equal restriction of all motions.

## Wrist Flexion

**Planes/axis of movement:** Motion occurs in the sagittal plane around a coronal axis primarily at the radiocarpal joint. Flexion also occurs at the midcarpal joint to a lesser degree, while the proximal row of carpal bones glide posteriorly on the distal end of the radius.

**Range of motion:**

- 0 degrees to 50 degrees (at the radiocarpal joint)
- 0 degrees to 35 degrees (at the midcarpal joint)
- 0 degrees to 90 degrees (from the anatomical position)

**Preferred starting position:** See Figure 2-44.

**End position:** See Figure 2-45.

**Goniometric alignment:**

- Axis: Center over the lateral aspect of the wrist, just distal to the styloid process of the ulna
- Stationary arm: Align with the lateral midline of the ulna, siting the olecranon process
- Moving arm: Align with the lateral midline of the fifth metacarpal bone

**Stabilization:** The forearm should be stabilized on a supporting surface.

**Substitutions:** The examiner must watch to make sure the forearm stays down on the table and the wrist does not drift into ulnar/radial deviation to avoid pain or gain more flexion.

**Alternate method/position for testing:** See Figure 2-46.

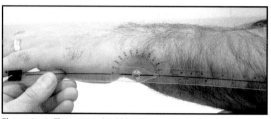

**Figure 2-44**. The patient should be sitting with the forearm resting on a table with the palm facing down. The shoulder should be abducted to 90 degrees with the elbow flexed to 90 degrees; the fingers should be loosely in extension.

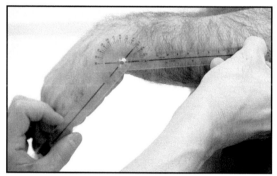

**Figure 2-45**. The wrist should be in a position of maximal flexion at the end of the movement.

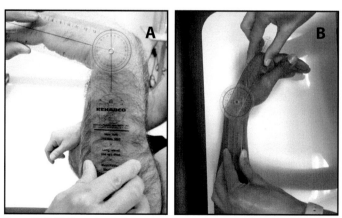

**Figure 2-46**. (A) The patient is sitting with the elbow flexed to 90 degrees with the olecranon process sitting on the table surface. The forearm is placed in a neutral position between pronation and supination. The fingers are held loosely in flexion. (B) The patient may also be placed in sitting with the forearm and wrist resting on a table top in a neutral position between pronation and supination. The fingers are held loosely in flexion.

GONIO

## Wrist Extension/Hyperextension

**Planes/axis of movement:** Motion occurs in the sagittal plane around a coronal axis at both the radiocarpal and midcarpal joint, with extension occurring more extensively at the latter.

**Range of motion:**

- 90 degrees to 0 degrees (from full flexion)
- 0 degrees to 70 degrees (hyperextension)

**Preferred starting position:** See Figure 2-47.

**End position:** See Figure 2-48.

**Goniometric alignment:**

- Axis: At the lateral aspect of the wrist, just distal to the ulnar styloid
- Stationary arm: Align with the lateral midline of the ulna, siting the olecranon process
- Moving arm: Align with the lateral midline of the fifth metacarpal bone

**Stabilization:** The forearm should be stabilized against a supporting surface.

**Substitutions:** The examiner should watch to make sure the forearm does not rise off the table or the wrist does not drift into ulnar/radial deviation to avoid a painful movement or to gain more extension.

**Alternate method/position for testing:** See Figure 2-49.

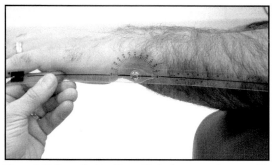

**Figure 2-47.** The patient is sitting with the forearm resting on a table with the palm facing down. The shoulder and elbow should be flexed to 90 degrees and the fingers should be held loosely in flexion.

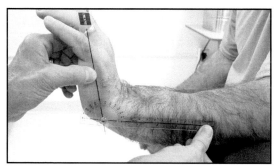

**Figure 2-48.** The wrist should be in a position of maximal extension/hyperextension at the end of the movement.

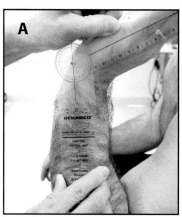
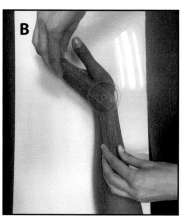

**Figure 2-49.** (A) The patient is sitting with the elbow flexed to 90 degrees with the olecranon process sitting on the table surface. The forearm is placed in a neutral position between pronation and supination. The fingers are held in extension. (B) The patient may also be placed in sitting with the forearm and wrist resting on a table top in a neutral position between pronation and supination. The fingers are held loosely in extension.

GONIO

# Wrist Radial Deviation (Abduction)

**Planes/axis of movement:** Motion occurs in the frontal/coronal plane in the anatomic position around an anterior/posterior axis. In the testing position, motion occurs in the transverse plane around a vertical axis. The motion occurs between the radiocarpal joint and the intercarpal bones.

**Range of motion:**

- 0 degrees to 25 degrees

**Preferred starting position:** See Figure 2-50.

**End position:** See Figure 2-51.

**Goniometric alignment:**

- Axis: Align over the middle of the dorsal surface of the wrist, over the capitate

- Stationary arm: Align with the dorsal midline of the forearm, siting the lateral epicondyle of the humerus

- Moving arm: Align with the midline of the dorsal surface of the third metacarpal

**Stabilization:** The distal ends of the radius and ulna must be stabilized against a supporting surface.

**Substitutions:** The patient may try to flex or extend the wrist or move the forearm into supination or pronation to avoid pain or gain more radial deviation.

**Alternate method/position for testing:** The patient may lie in supine if necessary with the palm facing down on the table.

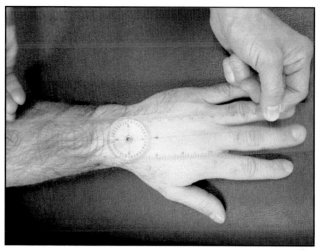

**Figure 2-50**. The patient is sitting with the shoulder abducted to 90 degrees and the elbow flexed to 90 degrees. The forearm rests on a supporting surface with the palm down. The wrist should be neutrally positioned between radial and ulnar deviation.

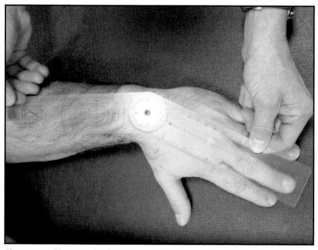

**Figure 2-51**. The wrist should be in a position of maximal radial deviation at the end of the movement.

# Wrist Ulnar Deviation (Adduction)

**Planes/axis of movement:** Motion occurs in the frontal/coronal plane in the anatomic position around an anterior/posterior axis. In the testing position, motion occurs in the transverse plane around a vertical axis. The motion occurs between the radiocarpal joint and the intercarpal bones.

**Range of motion:**

- 0 degrees to 35 degrees

**Preferred starting position:** See Figure 2-52.

**End position:** See Figure 2-53.

**Goniometric alignment:**

- Axis: Align the axis over the middle of the dorsal aspect of the wrist over the capitate

- Stationary arm: Align with the dorsal midline of the forearm, siting the lateral epicondyle of the humerus

- Moving arm: Align with the midline of the dorsal surface of the third metacarpal

**Stabilization:** The distal ends of the radius and ulna must be stabilized against a supporting surface.

**Substitutions:** The patient may try to flex or extend the wrist or move the forearm into supination or pronation to avoid pain or gain more ulnar deviation.

**Alternate method/position for testing:** The patient may lie in supine if necessary with the palm facing down on the table.

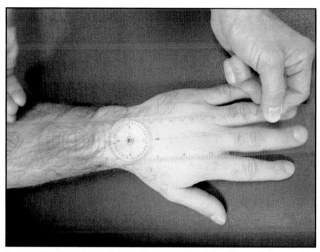

**Figure 2-52**. The patient is sitting with the shoulder abducted to 90 degrees and the elbow flexed to 90 degrees. The forearm rests on a supporting surface with the palm down. The wrist should be neutrally positioned between radial and ulnar deviation.

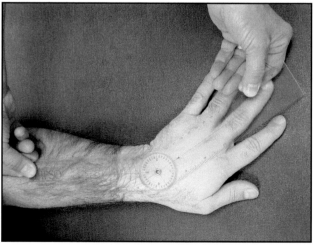

**Figure 2-53**. The wrist should be in a position of maximal ulnar deviation at the end of the movement.

# THE FINGERS— DIGITS II TO V (METACARPOPHALANGEAL JOINTS)

**Type of joint:** Condyloid, with the convex surfaces of the heads of the metacarpals articulating with the concave surfaces of the proximal phalanges.

**Capsular pattern:** Flexion > extension.

## MCP Flexion

**Planes/axis of movement:** Motion occurs in the sagittal plane around a transverse axis in the anatomical position, but in the testing position, motion occurs in the transverse plane around a vertical axis. Motion occurs between individual metacarpals and the corresponding phalanx, with the phalanx moving anteriorly on the metacarpal.

**Range of motion:**

- 0 degrees to 90 degrees of flexion (when moving with full extension of the interphalangeal joints)

**Preferred starting position:** See Figure 2-54.

**End position:** See Figure 2-55.

**Goniometric alignment:**

- Axis: Over the dorsal aspect of the metacarpophalangeal (MCP) joint
- Stationary arm: Align over the dorsal midline of the metacarpal bone
- Moving arm: Align over the dorsal midline of the proximal phalanx

**Stabilization:** The tested metacarpal must be stabilized to prevent wrist motion.

**Substitutions:** The patient may try to flex or deviate the wrist to avoid the movement because of pain.

**Alternate method/position for testing:** The patient may lie supine with the forearm lying in a neutral position on a supporting surface and with the wrist and fingers in a neutral position.

GONIO

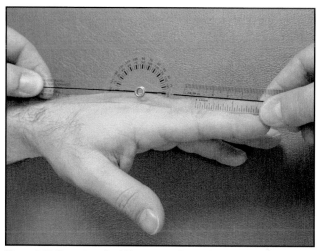

**Figure 2-54.** The patient should be sitting with the elbow in 90 degrees of flexion and the forearm should be in a neutral position between supination and pronation. The wrist and fingers should be in a neutral position.

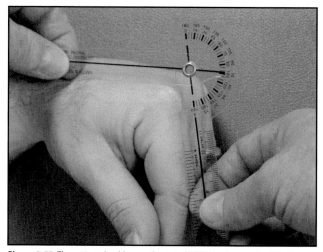

**Figure 2-55.** The patient should move the tested MCP joint into maximal flexion.

# MCP Extension/Hyperextension

**Planes/axis of movement:** Movement occurs in a transverse plane around a vertical axis when testing. Motion is considered hyperextension when it occurs beyond 0 degrees of extension.

**Range of motion:**

. 90 degrees to 0 degrees (extension)

. 0 degrees to 30 degrees (hyperextension)

**Preferred starting position:** See Figure 2-56.

**End position:** See Figure 2-57.

**Goniometric alignment:**

. Axis: Over the dorsal aspect of the MCP joint

. Stationary arm: Align over the dorsal midline of the metacarpal bone

. Moving arm: Align over the dorsal midline of the proximal phalanx

**Stabilization:** The tested metacarpal must be stabilized to prevent wrist motion.

**Substitutions:** The patient may try to deviate the wrist to avoid movement because of pain.

**Alternate method/position for testing:** See Figure 2-58.

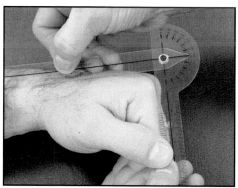

**Figure 2-56**. The patient should be sitting with the elbow in 90 degrees of flexion, with the forearm and wrist in neutral, and with the MCP joints in full flexion.

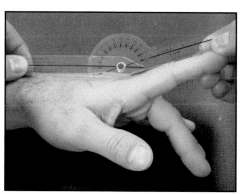

**Figure 2-57**. The patient should move the tested MCP joint into maximal extension/ hyperextension.

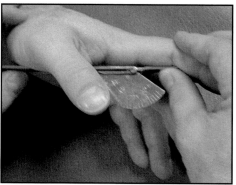

**Figure 2-58**. The goniometer may be placed on the palmar surface of the MCP joint to measure hyperextension.

# MCP Abduction

**Planes/axis of movement:** Motion occurs in the frontal plane around an anterior/posterior plane in the anatomical position. Motion occurs in the transverse plane around a vertical axis during testing. The second digit moves radially from the third digit, and the fourth and fifth digits move ulnarly from the middle finger.

**Range of motion:**

- 0 degrees to 20 degrees

**Preferred starting position:** See Figure 2-59.

**End position:** See Figure 2-60.

**Goniometric alignment:**

- Axis: Over the dorsal aspect of the MCP joint
- Stationary arm: Align over the dorsal midline of the metacarpal bone
- Moving arm: Align over the dorsal aspect of the proximal phalanx

**Stabilization:** The tested metacarpal must be stabilized to prevent wrist movement.

**Substitutions:** The patient may try to deviate the wrist into radial or ulnar deviation or into extension to avoid pain or gain motion with testing.

**Alternate method/position for testing:** The patient may lie supine with the elbow extended and the forearm lying in neutral on a supporting surface and with the wrist and fingers in neutral.

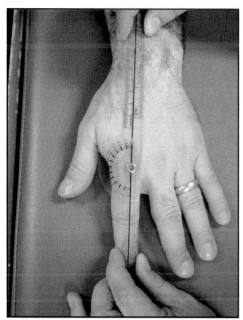

**Figure 2-59**. The patient should be sitting with the elbow flexed to 90 degrees and with the forearm in pronation with the palm facing the floor. The wrist should be in a neutral position between radial and ulnar deviation and the fingers should be extended.

GONIO

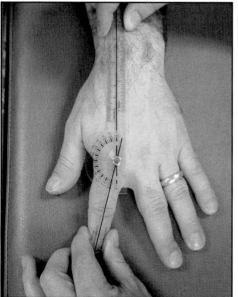

**Figure 2-60**. The patient should move the tested metacarpal into a position of maximal MCP abduction.

GONIO

# MCP Adduction

**Planes/axis of movement:** This is the return motion from MCP abduction. Motion occurs in the transverse plane around a vertical axis. The second digit moves in an ulnar direction, while the fourth and fifth digits move radially toward the middle finger.

**Range of motion:**

- 0 degrees to 20 degrees (with the middle finger positioned to allow for 20 degrees of motion to occur from the anatomical position)

**Preferred starting position:** See Figure 2-61.

**End position:** See Figure 2-62.

**Goniometric alignment:**

- Axis: Position over the dorsal aspect of the MCP joint

- Stationary arm: Align over the dorsal midline of the metacarpal bone

- Moving arm: Align over the dorsal aspect of the proximal phalanx

**Stabilization:** The tested metacarpal must be stabilized to prevent wrist movement.

**Substitutions:** The patient may try to deviate, flex, or extend the wrist to gain more movement or flex the MCP joints to gain more movement with testing.

**Alternate method/position for testing:** The patient may lie in supine with the elbow extended and with the forearm lying in neutral on a supporting surface, with the wrist and fingers in neutral.

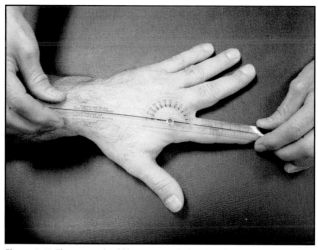

**Figure 2-61.** The patient should be sitting with the elbow flexed to 90 degrees and with the forearm in pronation with the palm facing the floor. The wrist should be in a neutral position between radial and ulnar deviation and the fingers should be extended.

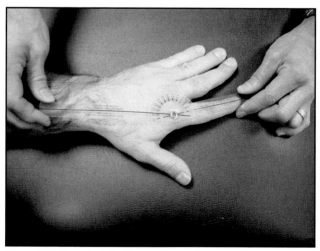

**Figure 2-62.** The patient should move the tested metacarpal into a position of maximal MCP adduction.

GONIO

# THE FINGERS— DIGITS II TO V (PROXIMAL INTERPHALANGEAL JOINTS)

**Type of joint:** Hinge joint with 1 degree of freedom, allowing only for flexion and extension.

**Capsular pattern:** Flexion > extension.

## PIP Flexion

**Planes/axis of movement:** In the testing position, movement occurs in the transverse plane around a vertical axis.

**Range of motion:**

- 0 degrees to 120 degrees

**Preferred starting position:** See Figure 2-63.

**End position:** See Figure 2-64.

**Goniometric alignment:**

- Axis: Over the dorsal aspect of the proximal interphalangeal (PIP) joint

- Stationary arm: Align over the dorsal midline of the proximal phalanx

- Moving arm: Align over the dorsal midline of the middle phalanx

**Stabilization:** The proximal phalanx should be stabilized to prevent motion at the MCP joint or wrist.

**Substitutions:** The patient may try to flex the wrist or MCP joint to avoid pain with the movement.

**Alternate method/position for testing:** None.

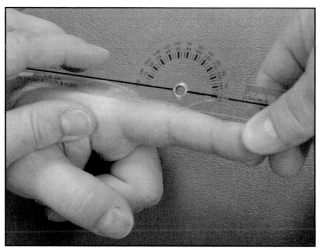

**Figure 2-63.** The patient should be in sitting with the forearm in neutral position and with the wrist and hand supported on a table top. The MCP, PIP, and distal interphalangeal (DIP) joints should be in a neutral position.

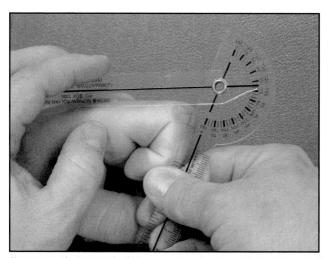

**Figure 2-64.** The PIP joint should be in a position of maximum flexion at the end of the movement.

GONIO

# PIP Extension

**Planes/axis of movement:** In the testing position, motion occurs in the transverse plane around a vertical axis.

**Range of motion:**

- 120 degrees to 0 degrees (from full flexion)
- 0 degrees to 10 degrees (hyperextension)

**Preferred starting position:** See Figure 2-65.

**End position:** See Figure 2-66.

**Goniometric alignment:**

- Axis: Over the dorsal aspect of the PIP joint
- Stationary arm: Align over the midline of the dorsal aspect of the proximal phalanx
- Moving arm: Align over the midline of the dorsal aspect of the middle phalanx

**Stabilization:** The proximal phalanx should be stabilized to prevent motion at the MCP joint or wrist.

**Substitutions:** The patient may try to extend the MCP joint or wrist to avoid pain or gain more movement during testing.

**Alternate method/position for testing:** See Figure 2-67.

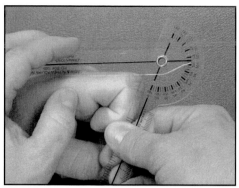

**Figure 2-65.** The patient should be in sitting with the forearm in neutral position and with the wrist and hand supported on a table top. The PIP and DIP joints should be in full flexion.

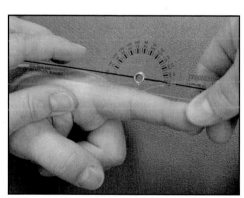

**Figure 2-66.** The PIP joint should be in a position of maximum extension/ hyperextension at the end of the movement.

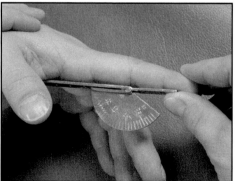

**Figure 2-67.** The goniometer may be placed on the palmar surface of the PIP joint to measure hyperextension.

**GONIO**

# THE FINGERS— DIGITS II TO V (DISTAL INTERPHALANGEAL JOINTS)

**Type of joint:** Hinge joint with 1 degree of freedom allowing only for flexion and extension.

**Capsular pattern:** Flexion > extension.

## DIP Flexion

**Planes/axis of movement:** In the testing position, motion occurs in the transverse plane around a vertical axis.

**Range of motion:**

- 0 degrees to 80 degrees

**Preferred starting position:** See Figure 2-68.

**End position:** See Figure 2-69.

**Goniometric alignment:**

- Axis: Over the dorsal aspect of the DIP joint
- Stationary arm: Align over the dorsal midline of the middle phalanx
- Moving arm: Align over the dorsal midline of the distal phalanx

**Stabilization:** The middle phalanx of the tested digit should be stabilized to prevent further flexion of the PIP and MCP joints.

**Substitutions:** The patient may try to slightly raise the forearm to avoid pain with movement.

**Alternate method/position for testing:** None.

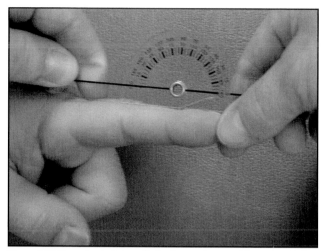

**Figure 2-68**. The patient is sitting with the elbow in flexion and the wrist and fingers in a neutral position, resting on a table top.

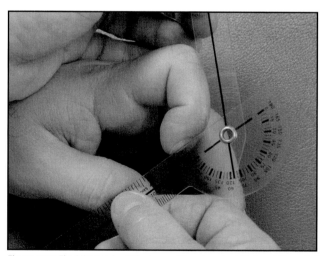

**Figure 2-69**. The DIP joint should be in a position of maximal flexion at the end of the movement.

# DIP Extension

**Planes/axis of movement:** In the testing position, motion occurs in a transverse plane around a vertical axis.

**Range of motion:**

- 80 degrees to 0 degrees (extension)
- 0 degrees to 10 degrees (hyperextension)

**Preferred starting position:** See Figure 2-70.

**End position:** See Figure 2-71.

**Goniometric alignment:**

- Axis: Over the dorsal aspect of the DIP joint
- Stationary arm: Align with the dorsal midline of the middle phalanx
- Moving arm: Align with the dorsal midline of the distal phalanx

**Stabilization:** The middle phalanx should be stabilized to prevent excessive extension of the PIP and MCP joints.

**Substitutions:** The patient may try to extend the PIP joint, MCP joint, or wrist to avoid pain with movement.

**Alternate method/position for testing:** See Figure 2-72.

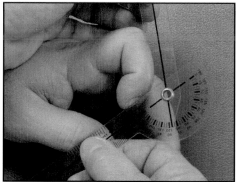

**Figure 2-70**. The patient should be sitting with the elbow flexed and the forearm and wrist in a neutral position resting on a table top. The PIP joint is flexed to approximately 80 degrees and the DIP joint should be in maximum flexion.

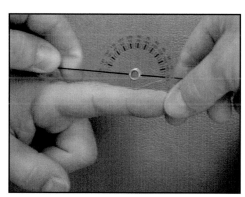

**Figure 2-71**. The DIP joint should be in a position of maximum extension at the end of the movement.

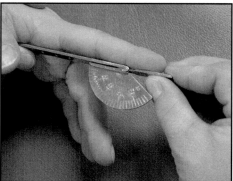

**Figure 2-72**. The goniometer may be placed on the palmar surface of the DIP joint to measure hyperextension.

# THE THUMB (CARPOMETACARPAL JOINT)

**Type of joint:** A saddle joint with multiple degrees of freedom, allowing for opposition and reposition of the thumb to occur.

**Capsular pattern:** Abduction > extension.

## CMC Flexion

**Planes/axis of movement:** Movement occurs in the frontal plane around an anterior/posterior axis in the anatomic position. In the testing position, movement occurs in the transverse plane around a vertical axis.

**Range of motion:**

- 0 degrees to 15 degrees

**Preferred starting position:** See Figure 2-73.

**End position:** See Figure 2-74.

**Goniometric alignment:**

- Axis: Center over the palmar aspect of the carpometacarpal (CMC) joint

- Stationary arm: Align over the palmar midline of the radial shaft

- Moving arm: Align over the palmar midline of the first metacarpal bone

> The goniometer arms may not align at 0 degrees in the start position, although the start position is recorded as such (ie, the start position may read 30 degrees). The range of motion for this movement is recorded as the total number of degrees between the start position and end position. Therefore, a measurement that begins with 30 degrees and ends at 15 degrees should be recorded as 0 to 15 degrees.

**Stabilization:** The forearm and wrist should be stabilized against a supporting surface to prevent wrist movement.

**Substitutions:** The patient may try to attempt to flex or ulnarly deviate the wrist to avoid the movement because of pain or to gain more motion. The examiner must also watch that the thumb does not move into opposition.

**Alternate method/position for testing:** None.

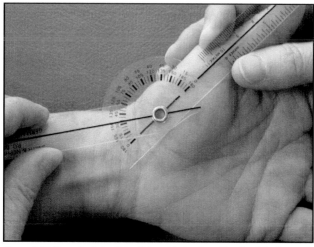

**Figure 2-73.** The patient should be sitting with the elbow flexed and the forearm in supination. The forearm and hand should rest on a table top. The wrist and MCP and interphalangeal (IP) joints of the thumb should be in a neutral position. The CMC joint should be in midposition between abduction and adduction.

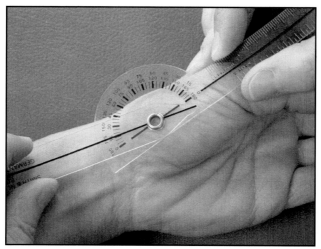

**Figure 2-74.** The CMC joint of the thumb should be maximally flexed at the end of the motion.

# CMC Extension

**Planes/axis of movement:** Movement occurs in the frontal plane around an anterior/posterior axis in the anatomic position. In the testing position, movement occurs in the transverse plane around a vertical axis.

**Range of motion:**

- 0 degrees to 20 degrees

**Preferred starting position:** See Figure 2-75.

**End position:** See Figure 2-76.

**Goniometric alignment:**

- Axis: Center over the palmar aspect of the CMC joint

- Stationary arm: Align over the palmar midline of the radius

- Moving arm: Align over the palmar midline of the first metacarpal bone

> The goniometer arms may not align at 0 degrees in the start position, although the start position is recorded as such (ie, the start position may read 30 degrees). The range of motion for this movement is recorded as the total number of degrees between the start and end position. Therefore, a measurement that begins with 30 degrees and ends at 50 degrees should be recorded as 0 to 20 degrees.

**Stabilization:** The forearm and wrist must be stabilized against a supporting surface to prevent wrist movement.

**Substitutions:** The patient may try to extend or radially deviate the wrist to increase the motion or avoid pain. The patient may also abduct the thumb to avoid pain.

**Alternate method/position for testing:** None.

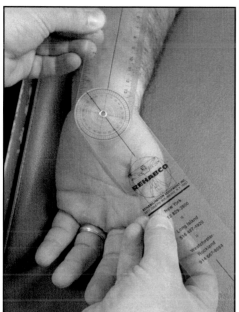

**Figure 2-75**. The patient should be sitting with the elbow flexed and the forearm in supination. The forearm and hand should rest on a table top. The wrist and MCP and IP joints of the thumb should be in a neutral position. The CMC joint should be in midposition between abduction and adduction.

GONIO

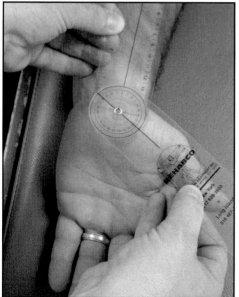

**Figure 2-76**. The CMC joint of the thumb should be maximally extended at the end of the movement.

**GONIO**

# CMC Abduction

**Planes/axis of movement:** During testing, motion occurs in a transverse plane around a vertical axis. The thumb moves at a right angle to the palm.

**Range of motion:**

- 0 degrees to 60 degrees

**Preferred starting position:** See Figure 2-77.

**End position:** See Figure 2-78.

**Goniometric alignment:**

- Axis: Center over the dorsal aspect of the CMC joint

- Stationary arm: Align with the lateral midline of the second metacarpal bone

- Moving arm: Align with the lateral midline of the first metacarpal bone

> The goniometer arms may not align at 0 degrees in the start position, although the start position is recorded as such (ie, the start position may read 15 to 20 degrees). The range of motion for this movement is recorded as the total number of degrees between the start and end position. Therefore, a measurement that begins at 15 degrees and ends at 60 degrees should be recorded as 45 degrees of CMC abduction.

**Stabilization:** The wrist and second metacarpal should be stabilized against a supporting surface to prevent wrist movement.

**Substitutions:** The patient may try to flex or extend the wrist or oppose the thumb to increase movement or to avoid pain during testing.

**Alternate method/position for testing:** None.

GONIO

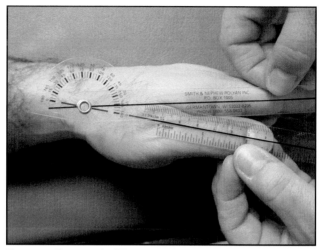

**Figure 2-77**. The patient should be sitting with the elbow flexed and the forearm and wrist in a neutral position resting on a table top. The CMC, MCP, and IP joints should be in a neutral position between flexion and extension.

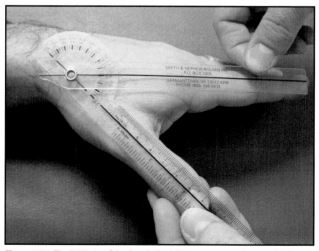

**Figure 2-78**. The CMC joint of the thumb should be in a position of maximal abduction at the end of the movement.

# CMC Adduction

**Planes/axis of movement:** During testing, motion occurs in a transverse plane around a vertical axis.

**Range of motion:**

- 60 degrees to 0 degrees

**Preferred starting position:** See Figure 2-79.

**End position:** See Figure 2-80.

**Goniometric alignment:**

- Axis: Center over the dorsal aspect of the CMC joint
- Stationary arm: Align with the lateral midline of the second metacarpal bone
- Moving arm: Align with the lateral midline of the first metacarpal bone

> The goniometer arms will not align at 0 degrees at the start position, although the start position is recorded as such (ie, the start position may read 60 degrees). The range of motion for this movement is recorded as the total number of degrees between the start and end position. Therefore, a measurement that begins at 60 degrees and ends at 15 degrees should be recorded as 45 degrees of CMC adduction.

**Stabilization:** The wrist and second metacarpal should be stabilized against a supporting surface to prevent wrist movement.

**Substitutions:** The patient may try to flex, extend, or oppose the thumb to increase movement or to avoid pain during testing.

**Alternate method/position for testing:** None.

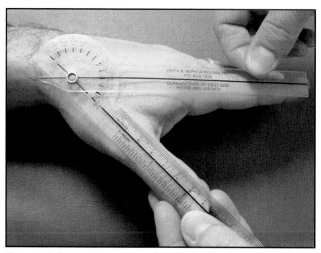

**Figure 2-79.** The patient should be sitting with the elbow flexed and the forearm and wrist in a neutral position resting on a table top. The CMC should be in full abduction and the MCP and IP joints should be in a neutral position between flexion and extension.

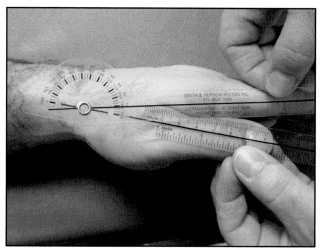

**Figure 2-80.** The CMC joint of the thumb should be in a position of maximal adduction at the end of the movement.

## CMC Opposition

**Planes/axis of movement:** This motion combines the movements of flexion, abduction, and internal rotation of the first metacarpal and trapezium. The thumb moves toward the tip of the fifth digit with the pad of the thumb touching the pad of the fifth digit. It moves through a varying array of planes and axes.

**Range of motion:**

- Variable, "normal" range of motion allows for complete motion until the tips of the thumb and fifth digit meet from an open-palm position

**Preferred starting position:** See Figure 2-81.

**End position:** See Figure 2-82.

**Goniometric alignment:**

- In this motion, a ruler is used in place of a goniometer to record the deficit of complete range of motion; the ruler is placed from the tip of the thumb to the tip of the fifth digit

**Stabilization:** The fifth metacarpal should be stabilized against a supporting surface to prevent wrist movement.

**Substitutions:** The patient may try to attempt to flex the wrist to increase the motion.

**Alternate method/position for testing:** None.

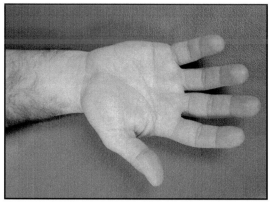

**Figure 2-81**. The patient is sitting with the elbow flexed and the forearm supported in a fully supinated position. The wrist is in a neutral position and the IP joint of the thumb and fifth digit are in a neutral position between flexion and extension.

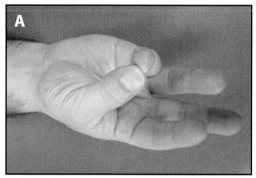

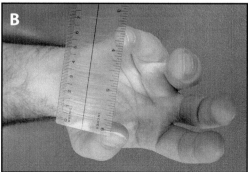

**Figure 2-82**. The thumb should be maximally opposed at the end of the movement. (A) Full CMC opposition. (B) CMC opposition deficit.

# THE THUMB (METACARPOPHALANGEAL JOINT)

**Type of joint:** Hinge joint that allows for 1 degree of freedom in flexion and extension.

**Capsular pattern:** Flexion > extension.

## MCP Flexion

**Planes/axis of movement:** Movement occurs in the transverse plane around a vertical axis during testing.

**Range of motion:**

- 0 degrees to 50 degrees

**Preferred starting position:** See Figure 2-83.

**End position:** See Figure 2-84.

**Goniometric alignment:**

- Axis: Center over the dorsal aspect of the MCP joint
- Stationary arm: Align over the dorsal midline of the first metacarpal bone
- Moving arm: Align over the dorsal midline of the proximal phalanx

**Stabilization:** The first metacarpal and CMC joint of the thumb should be stabilized.

**Substitutions:** The patient may try to flex the wrist to increase the movement or avoid pain during testing.

**Alternate method/position for testing:** None.

GONIO

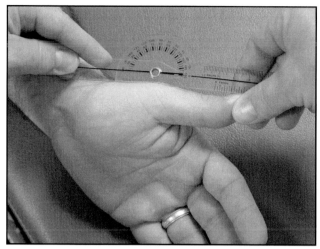

**Figure 2-83**. The patient is in sitting with the elbow flexed. The forearm should be in supination with the wrist in a neutral position. The CMC and IP joints should be in a neutral position. The forearm, wrist, and hand should be resting on a table top.

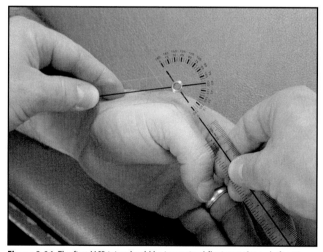

**Figure 2-84**. The first MCP joint should be in maximal flexion at the end of testing.

# MCP Extension/Hyperextension

**Planes/axis of movement:** This motion is the return movement from thumb MCP flexion. This movement occurs in the transverse plane around a vertical axis during testing.

**Range of motion:**

- 50 degrees to 0 degrees (extension)
- 0 degrees to 10 degrees (hyperextension)

**Preferred starting position:** See Figure 2-85.

**End position:** See Figure 2-86.

**Goniometric alignment:**

- Axis: Center over the dorsal surface of the MCP joint
- Stationary arm: Align along the dorsal surface of the first metacarpal bone
- Moving arm: Align along the dorsal midline of the proximal phalanx of the thumb

**Stabilization:** The first metacarpal and CMC joint of the thumb should be stabilized.

**Substitutions:** The patient may try to flex or radially deviate the wrist to gain more motion or avoid pain during movement.

**Alternate method/position for testing:** See Figure 2-87.

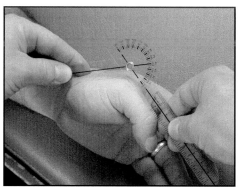

**Figure 2-85**. The patient is sitting with the elbow flexed, the forearm in supination, and with the wrist and fingers in a neutral position. The first MCP joint should be in full flexion. The forearm, wrist, and hand should be resting on a table top.

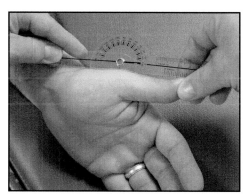

**Figure 2-86**. The first MCP joint should be in maximal extension at the end of the movement.

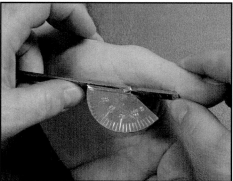

**Figure 2-87**. The goniometer may be placed on the palmar surface of the MCP joint to measure hyperextension.

# THE THUMB (INTERPHALANGEAL JOINT)

**Type of joint:** Hinge joint with 1 degree of freedom allowing only for flexion and extension.

**Capsular pattern:** Flexion > extension.

## IP Flexion

**Planes/axis of movement:** Movement occurs in the transverse plane around a vertical axis during testing.

**Range of motion:**

- 0 degrees to 90 degrees

**Preferred starting position:** See Figure 2-88.

**End position:** See Figure 2-89.

**Goniometric alignment:**

- Axis: Center over the dorsal surface of the IP joint
- Stationary arm: Align with the dorsal midline of the proximal phalanx
- Moving arm: Align with the dorsal midline of the distal phalanx

**Stabilization:** The proximal phalanx of the thumb should be stabilized.

**Substitutions:** The patient may try to flex the wrist or first MCP joint to increase the amount of the range of motion or avoid pain during testing.

**Alternate method/position for testing:** None.

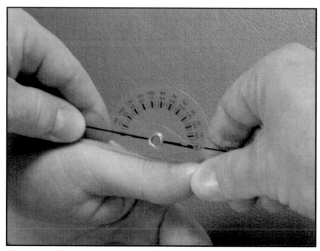

**Figure 2-88**. The patient is sitting with the elbow flexed and the forearm in full supination. The wrist and CMC joints of the thumb should be in a neutral position. The forearm and hand should rest on a table top.

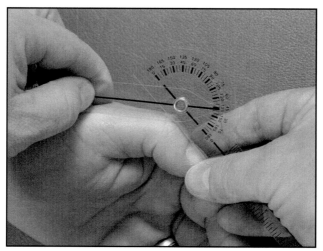

**Figure 2-89**. The IP joint of the thumb should be maximally flexed at the end of the movement.

## IP Extension/Hyperextension

**Planes/axis of movement:** Movement occurs in the transverse plane around a vertical axis during testing. This is the return motion from full thumb IP flexion.

**Range of motion:**

- 90 degrees to 0 degrees

**Preferred starting position:** See Figure 2-90.

**End position:** See Figure 2-91.

**Goniometric alignment:**

- Axis: Center over the dorsal aspect of the IP joint
- Stationary arm: Align over the dorsal midline of the proximal phalanx
- Moving arm: Align over the dorsal midline of the distal phalanx

**Stabilization:** The proximal phalanx of the thumb should be stabilized.

**Substitutions:** The patient may try to extend the wrist, CMC joint, or first MCP joint to increase the range of motion during testing.

**Alternate method/position for testing:** See Figure 2-92.

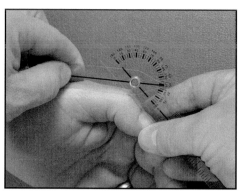

**Figure 2-90**. The patient is in sitting with the elbow flexed and the forearm fully supinated. The wrist, CMC joint, and MCP joint of the thumb should be in a neutral position with the IP joint in full flexion.

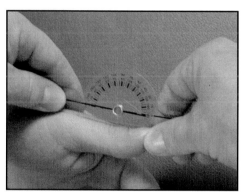

**Figure 2-91**. The IP joint of the thumb should be in maximal extension at the end of the movement.

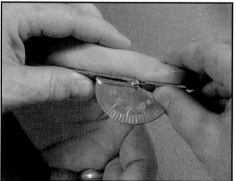

**Figure 2-92**. The goniometer may be placed on the palmar surface of the IP joint to measure hyperextension.

GONIO

# SECTION III
# Thoracic and Lumbar Spine

Van Ost L, Morogiello J.
*Cram Session in Goniometry and Manual Muscle Testing:
A Handbook for Students & Clinicians, Second Edition* (pp 89-97).
© 2023 Taylor & Francis Group.

# THE THORACOLUMBAR SPINE

**Type of joint:** The thoracic and lumbar spine are very complex structures involving segmented movement at numerous vertebral articulations. As a result, it is not possible to accurately measure all movements occurring along this area of the spine with a goniometer. An alternative method will be addressed.

**Capsular pattern:** Lateral flexion = rotation/extension.

## Thoracolumbar Flexion

**Planes/axis of movement:** Movement occurs in the sagittal plane around a coronal axis.

**Range of motion:**

- Approximately 4-inch difference between initial and ending measurements

**Preferred starting position:** See Figure 3-1.

**End position:** See Figure 3-2.

**Measurement of motion:** The distance between the spinous processes of C7 and S1 is first measured in standing. The patient then flexes the trunk as far forward as possible and the second measurement is taken. The difference between the 2 measurements is the amount of flexion present.

**Stabilization:** The pelvis should be stabilized to prevent anterior tilting. Stabilization is achieved through patient compliance.

**Substitutions:** See Figure 3-3.

**Alternate method/position for testing:** None.

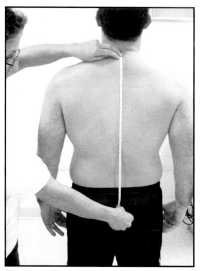

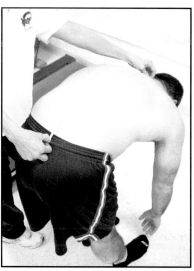

**Figure 3-1**. The patient should be standing in an erect position with the arms by the sides.

**Figure 3-2**. The thoracolumbar spine is maximally flexed forward.

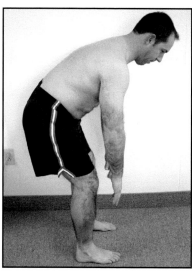

**Figure 3-3**. The patient may try to flex the hips and/or the knees during movement to gain more flexion. This may occur as the hamstrings are maximally stretched.

# Thoracolumbar Extension/ Hyperextension

**Planes/axis of movement:** Extension is the return motion from full thoracolumbar flexion. Beyond 0 degrees starting position is considered hyperextension. Motion occurs in the sagittal plane around a coronal axis.

**Range of motion:**

- Approximately 2-inch difference between the initial and ending measurements

**Preferred starting position:** See Figure 3-4.

**End position:** See Figure 3-5.

**Measurement of motion:** The distance between the spinous processes of C7 and S1 is first measured in standing. The patient extends the trunk as far backward as possible and a second measurement is taken. The difference between the 2 measurements is the amount of extension present.

**Stabilization:** The pelvis should be stabilized to prevent posterior tilting. Stabilization is achieved through patient compliance.

**Substitutions:** See Figure 3-6.

**Alternate method/position for testing:** None.

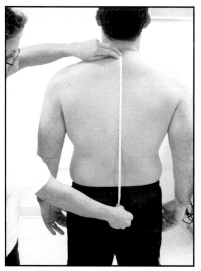 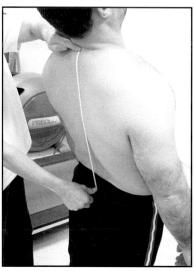

**Figure 3-4**. The patient should be standing in an erect position with the arms by the sides.

**Figure 3-5**. The thoracolumbar spine is maximally extended at the end of the motion.

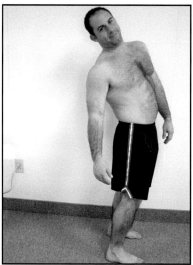

**Figure 3-6**. The patient may try to laterally bend or rotate the trunk during testing to gain more motion or avoid pain. The patient may also bend the knees as the hip flexors are maximally stretched.

# Thoracolumbar Lateral Flexion

**Planes/axis of movement:** Motion occurs in the frontal plane around an anterior/posterior axis.

**Range of motion:**

- Range of motion is variable because of the differences in arm and trunk length; the amount of motion is determined by the comparison of both sides

**Preferred starting position:** See Figure 3-7.

**End position:** See Figure 3-8.

**Measurement of motion:** The distance between the tip of the middle finger and floor is taken first. The patient then laterally flexes to the side as far as possible and a second measurement is taken. The difference between the 2 measurements is the amount of lateral flexion present.

**Stabilization:** The pelvis should be stabilized during testing. Stabilization is achieved through patient compliance.

**Substitutions:** See Figure 3-9.

**Alternate method/position for testing:** None.

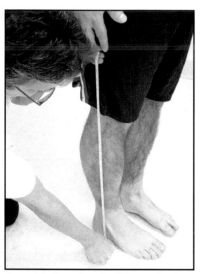

**Figure 3-7**. The patient should be standing in an erect position with the arms by the sides.

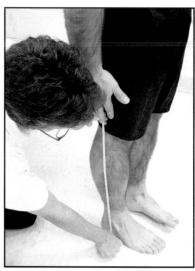

**Figure 3-8**. The thoracolumbar spine is maximally laterally flexed to the tested side.

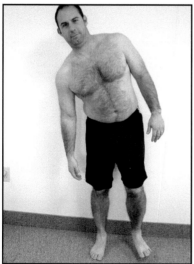

**Figure 3-9**. The patient may try to flex, extend, or rotate the trunk during testing or lift the opposite lower extremity off the floor to gain more motion.

# Thoracolumbar Rotation

**Planes/axis of movement:** Motion occurs in the transverse plane around a vertical axis.

**Range of motion:**

- 0 degrees to 45 degrees

**Preferred starting position:** See Figure 3-10.

**End position:** See Figure 3-11.

**Goniometric alignment:**

- Axis: Align over the center of the top of the head

- Stationary arm: Align parallel to an imaginary line between the 2 iliac crests

- Moving arm: Align parallel to the top of the shoulder, siting the acromion process

**Stabilization:** The pelvis should be stabilized during testing. Stabilization is achieved through patient compliance.

**Substitutions:** The patient may try to flex, extend, or laterally flex the trunk to increase the motion. They may also try to raise the pelvis.

**Alternate method/position for testing:** None.

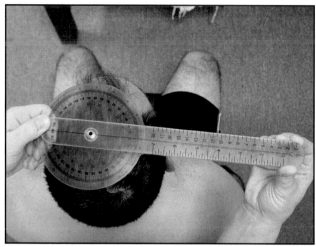

**Figure 3-10**. Preferably, the patient should be sitting without a back support to ensure full mobility. The cervical, thoracic, and lumbar spine should be in a neutral position with the arms resting by the sides.

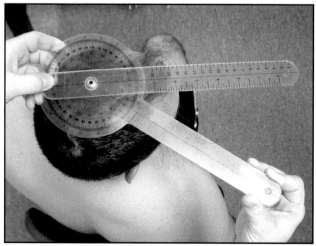

**Figure 3-11**. The thorax should be maximally rotated to the tested side at the end of the movement.

# SECTION IV

# Lower Extremity

Van Ost L, Morogiello J.
*Cram Session in Goniometry and Manual Muscle Testing:*
*A Handbook for Students & Clinicians, Second Edition* (pp 99-151).
© 2023 Taylor & Francis Group.

GONIO

# THE HIP

**Type of joint:** Ball and socket joint with 3 degrees of freedom.

**Capsular pattern:** Internal/external rotation > abduction > flexion > extension > adduction.

## Hip Flexion

**Planes/axis of movement:** Motion occurs in the sagittal plane around a coronal axis. During testing, the knee is allowed to flex passively so the hamstrings do not limit movement.

**Range of motion:**

- 0 degrees to 115 degrees (with the knee extended)
- 0 degrees to 125 degrees (with the knee flexed)

**Preferred starting position:** See Figure 4-1.

**End position:** See Figure 4-2.

**Goniometric alignment:**

- Axis: Center on the lateral aspect of the hip joint over the greater trochanter of the femur
- Stationary arm: Align parallel to the lateral midline of the trunk
- Moving arm: Align parallel to the lateral midline of the femur, siting the lateral epicondyle

**Stabilization:** The pelvis should be stabilized against a supporting surface by the weight of the body.

**Substitutions:** The patient may try to flex the lumbar spine or opposite hip during testing.

**Alternate method/position for testing:** See Figure 4-3.

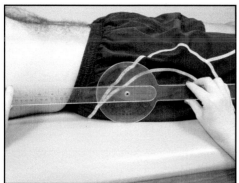

**Figure 4-1**. The patient lies supine with the hip in midposition between abduction, adduction, and rotation. The opposite lower extremity is extended and rests on a supporting surface.

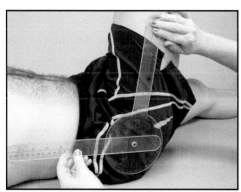

**Figure 4-2**. The hip should be in a position of maximum hip flexion at the end of the movement.

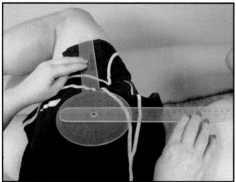

**Figure 4-3**. The patient may be positioned in sidelying on the uninvolved side.

# Hip Extension/Hyperextension

**Planes/axis of movement:** Movement occurs in the sagittal plane around a coronal axis. Extension and hyperextension are the "return" movements from a position of hip flexion.

**Range of motion:**

- 125 degrees to 0 degrees (extension)

- 0 degrees to 15 degrees (hyperextension)

**Preferred starting position:** See Figure 4-4.

**End position:** See Figure 4-5.

**Goniometric alignment:**

- Axis: Center on the lateral aspect of the hip joint over the greater trochanter of the femur

- Stationary arm: Align parallel to the lateral midline of the trunk

- Moving arm: Align parallel to the lateral midline of the femur, siting the lateral epicondyle

**Stabilization:** The pelvis should be stabilized against a supporting surface by the weight of the body, a strap, or the clinician's hand if necessary.

**Substitutions:** The patient may try to extend the lumbar spine or rotate the hips to avoid pain or increase the motion.

**Alternate method/position for testing:** The patient may be positioned in sidelying on the uninvolved side. The nontested hip should be flexed to 90 degrees to prevent anterior pelvic tilting.

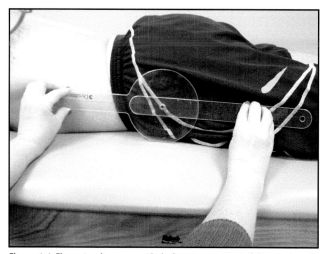

**Figure 4-4**. The patient lies prone with the lower extremities in full extension with both hips in a neutral position.

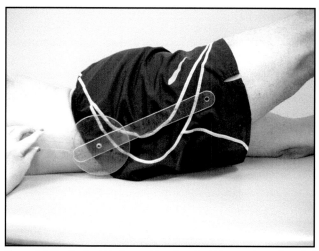

**Figure 4-5**. The hip should be in a position of maximal hip extension at the end of the movement.

# Hip Abduction

**Planes/axis of movement:** Movement occurs in a frontal plane around an anterior/posterior axis.

**Range of motion:**

- 0 degrees to 45 degrees

**Preferred starting position:** See Figure 4-6.

**End position:** See Figure 4-7.

**Goniometric alignment:**

- Axis: Center over the anterior aspect of the hip joint at the anterior superior iliac spine (ASIS)
- Stationary arm: Align with an imaginary horizontal line, siting the ASIS of the opposite hip
- Moving arm: Align with the anterior midline of the femur, siting the center of the patella

**Stabilization:** The pelvis should be stabilized against a supporting surface. The clinician may use their hand on the lateral aspect of the knee to prevent hip rotation.

**Substitutions:** The patient may try to rotate the tested hip or bend laterally to the opposite side to increase the motion or avoid pain. They may also try to tilt the pelvis on the contralateral side.

**Alternate method/position for testing:** None.

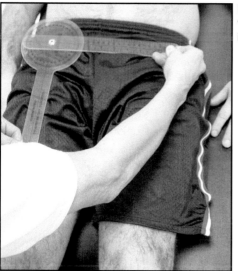

**Figure 4-6.** The patient should lie supine with the hip in midposition between flexion/extension and rotation.

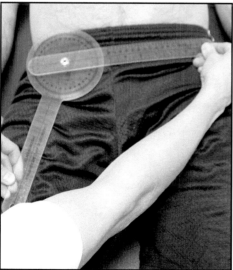

**Figure 4-7**. The hip should be in a position of maximal abduction at the end of the movement.

# Hip Adduction

**Planes/axis of movement:** Movement occurs in the frontal plane around an anterior/posterior axis. This is the return motion from abduction.

**Range of motion:**

- 0 degrees to 30 degrees

**Preferred starting position:** See Figure 4-8.

**End position:** See Figure 4-9.

**Goniometric alignment:**

- Axis: Center over the anterior aspect of the hip joint at the ASIS

- Stationary arm: Align with an imaginary horizontal line, siting the ASIS of the opposite hip

- Moving arm: Align with the anterior midline of the femur, siting the center of the patella

**Stabilization:** The pelvis should be stabilized against a supporting surface and encourage patient compliance to prevent ipsilateral tilting of the pelvis.

**Substitutions:** The patient may try to attempt to laterally flex the trunk toward the tested side to increase the range of motion or avoid pain with movement.

**Alternate method/position for testing:** None.

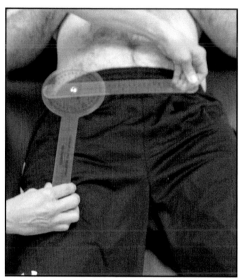

**Figure 4-8.** The patient lies in supine with the opposite lower extremity fully abducted to allow for full adduction of the tested limb. The hip should be in a neutral position between flexion/extension and rotation. The knee should be extended.

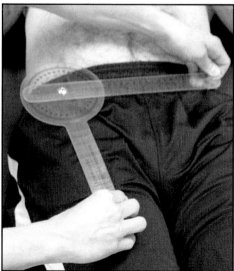

**Figure 4-9.** The tested hip should be in a position of maximal adduction at the end of the movement.

GONIO

# Hip Internal (Medial) Rotation

**Planes/axis of movement:** Movement occurs in the transverse plane around a longitudinal axis in the anatomic position and in the frontal plane around an anterior/posterior axis during testing.

**Range of motion:**

- 0 degrees to 45 degrees (with the hip flexed)

- 0 degrees to 30 degrees (with the hip extended)

**Preferred starting position:** See Figure 4-10.

**End position:** See Figure 4-11.

**Goniometric alignment:**

- Axis: Center over the midpatellar surface

- Stationary arm: Align so the goniometer is perpendicular to the floor or parallel to the table top

- Moving arm: Align with the anterior midline of the lower leg, siting the midpoint between the 2 malleoli of the ankle

**Stabilization:** The distal end of the femur should be stabilized against a supporting surface through body weight. The clinician may have to use their hand to prevent hip adduction or flexion.

**Substitutions:** The patient may try to tilt the pelvis on the contralateral side or raise the pelvis off the table to increase the range of motion. They may also adduct the hip to avoid pain.

**Alternate method/position for testing:** See Figure 4-12.

GONIO

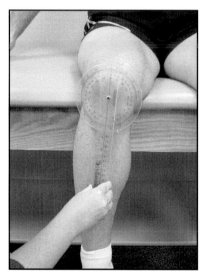

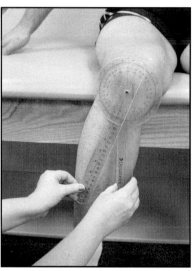

**Figure 4-10**. The patient should be in sitting on a table top with the hips and knees flexed to 90 degrees. The lower limb should hang freely over the edge of the table.

**Figure 4-11**. The hips should be in a position of maximal internal rotation at the end of the movement.

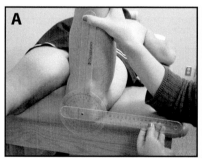

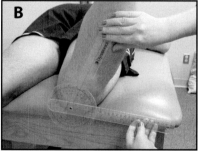

**Figure 4-12**. The patient may lie prone or supine with the hip in a neutral position with the knee flexed to 90 degrees. (A) Alternate starting position. (B) End position.

# Hip External (Lateral) Rotation

**Planes/axis of movement:** Movement occurs in the transverse plane around a longitudinal axis in the anatomic position and in a frontal plane around an anterior/posterior axis during testing.

**Range of motion:**

- 0 degrees to 45 degrees (with the hip flexed)

- 0 degrees to 30 degrees (with the hip extended)

**Preferred starting position:** See Figure 4-13.

**End position:** See Figure 4-14.

**Goniometric alignment:**

- Axis: Center over the anterior midpatellar surface

- Stationary arm: Align so the goniometer is perpendicular to the floor or parallel to the table top

- Moving arm: Align with the anterior midline of the lower leg, siting the midpoint between the 2 malleoli of the ankle

**Stabilization:** The distal end of the femur should be stabilized against a supporting surface through body weight. The clinician may have to use their hand to prevent hip abduction or flexion.

**Substitutions:** See Figure 4-15.

**Alternate method/position for testing:** The patient may lie supine or prone with the hip in neutral with the knee flexed to 90 degrees.

GONIO

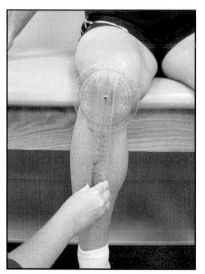

**Figure 4-13.** The patient should be sitting on a table top with the hips and knees flexed to 90 degrees. The lower limb should hang freely over the edge of the table.

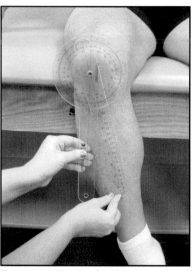

**Figure 4-14.** The hip should be in a position of maximal external rotation at the end of the movement.

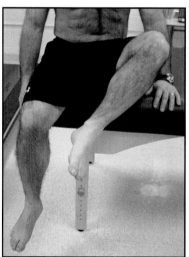

**Figure 4-15.** The patient may try to tilt or rotate the pelvis toward the ipsilateral side or raise the pelvis off the table to gain more range of motion. They may also try to abduct or flex the hip to avoid pain with movement.

# THE KNEE
# (TIBIOFEMORAL JOINT)

**Type of joint:** The knee is a hinge joint with 2 degrees of freedom, allowing for flexion and extension with an axial rotation.

**Capsular pattern:** Flexion > extension.

## Knee Flexion

**Planes/axis of movement:** Motion occurs in the sagittal plane around a coronal axis. Axial rotation occurs in the transverse plane when the knee is in a flexed position.

**Range of motion:**

- 0 degrees to 120 degrees (with the hip extended)
- 0 degrees to 135 degrees (with the hip flexed)

**Preferred starting position:** See Figure 4-16.

**End position:** See Figure 4-17.

**Goniometric alignment:**

- Axis: Center over the lateral epicondyle of the femur
- Stationary arm: Align with the lateral midline of the femur, siting the greater trochanter
- Moving arm: Align with the lateral midline of the fibula, siting the lateral malleolus

**Stabilization:** The pelvis should be stabilized against a supporting surface and the femur should be stabilized by the clinician's hand if necessary to prevent any hip movement.

**Substitutions:** The patient may try to rotate the hip to avoid pain.

**Alternate method/position for testing:** See Figure 4-18.

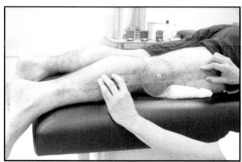

**Figure 4-16**. The patient is placed in prone with the hip in neutral position. The foot should be placed over the edge of the table top. A folded towel should be placed under the anterior thigh to prevent compression on the patella.

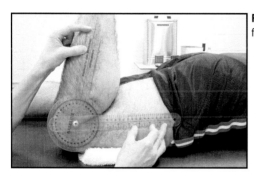

**Figure 4-17**. The knee should be maximally flexed at the end of the movement.

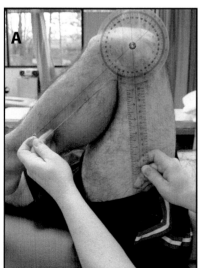
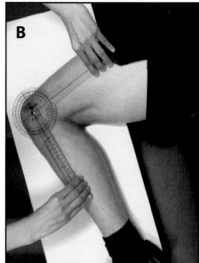

**Figure 4-18**. (A) The patient may be placed supine with the hip flexed to 90 degrees or the patient may be placed in sidelying with the leg to be tested on the top. The knee and hip are both flexed in this position. (B) The patient may be placed in sidelying with a slide board between the legs.

# Knee Extension

**Planes/axis of movement:** Motion occurs in the sagittal plane around a coronal axis. Extension is the return motion from knee flexion.

**Range of motion:**

- 120 degrees to 0 degrees (from knee flexion with the hip extended)
- 135 degrees to 0 degrees (from knee flexion with the hip flexed)

**Preferred starting position:** See Figure 4-19.

**End position:** See Figure 4-20.

**Goniometric alignment:**

- Axis: Center over the lateral epicondyle of the femur
- Stationary arm: Align with the lateral midline of the femur, siting the greater trochanter
- Moving arm: Align with the lateral midline of the fibula, siting the lateral malleolus

**Stabilization:** The pelvis should be stabilized against a supporting surface and the femur should be stabilized by the clinician's hand if necessary to prevent any hip movement.

**Substitutions:** The patient may try to rotate the hip to avoid pain with movement.

**Alternate method/position for testing:** The patient may be placed in sidelying with the leg to be tested on top.

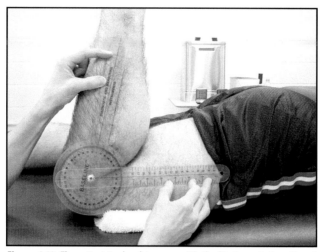

**Figure 4-19**. The patient is placed in prone with the hip in neutral position. A folded towel should be placed under the anterior thigh to prevent compression on the patella. The knee joint should be in a maximally flexed position.

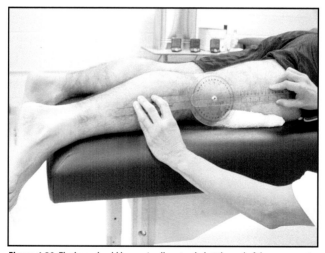

**Figure 4-20**. The knee should be maximally extended at the end of the movement.

# TIBIAL TORSION

Tibial torsion is described as a slight lateral angulation of the distal tibia in comparison to the proximal aspect of the tibia. It may be assessed with a goniometer by measuring the angle of the malleoli to the talus.

**Range of motion:**

- 20 degrees to 30 degrees of torsion

**Preferred starting position:** See Figure 4-21 (in supine) and Figure 4-22 (in prone).

**End position:** See Figure 4-21 (in supine) and Figure 4-22 (in prone).

**Goniometric alignment:** A line should be drawn on the bottom of the heel horizontal to the table top. A second line is drawn on the bottom of the heel in line with both malleoli.

- Axis: Center over the intersection of the 2 lines
- Stationary arm: Align parallel to the table top in line with the horizontal line on the heel
- Moving arm: Align along the line connecting the 2 malleoli

**Stabilization:** The lower leg should be stabilized on a supporting surface.

**Substitutions:** The patient may move the lower limb during testing, which may cause an inaccurate measurement to be taken.

**Alternate method/position for testing:** The patient lies in prone with the knee flexed to 90 degrees.

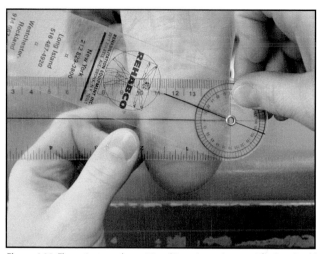

**Figure 4-21**. The patient may be positioned in supine or in prone. The foot should rest over the edge of the table top. The ankle and foot should be in a neutral position. The position remains the same throughout the measurement. Measurement shown in supine.

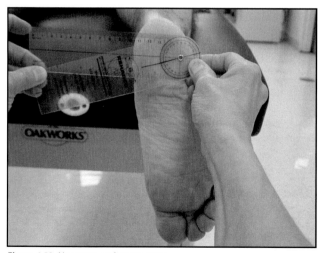

**Figure 4-22**. Measurement shown in prone.

# THE ANKLE

**Type of joint:** Hinge joint with 1 degree of freedom. The axis of motion is obliquely oriented in the transverse plane and passes along a line that connects 2 points just distal to the tips of the malleoli. The movements of plantarflexion and dorsiflexion occur at this joint.

**Capsular pattern:** Plantarflexion > dorsiflexion.

## Ankle Dorsiflexion

**Planes/axis of movement:** Motion occurs in the sagittal plane around a coronal axis.

**Range of motion:**

- 0 degrees to 20 degrees

**Preferred starting position:** See Figure 4-23.

**End position:** See Figure 4-24.

**Goniometric alignment:**

- Axis: Center over the lateral aspect of the lateral malleolus
- Stationary arm: Align with the lateral midline of the fibula, siting the fibular head
- Moving arm: Align with the lateral midline of the calcaneus

**Stabilization:** The tibia and fibula must be stabilized by the clinician (or on a supporting surface if the patient is in supine or prone) to prevent hip or knee motion.

**Substitutions:** The patient may try to flex the knee or hip to gain more range of motion or avoid pain during testing.

**Alternate method/position for testing:** See Figure 4-25.

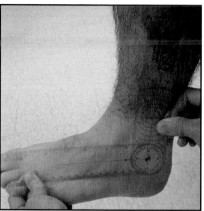

**Figure 4-23**. The patient is in sitting or supine with the knee flexed to at least 30 degrees. The foot should be in midposition between inversion and eversion. A towel roll is placed under the knee to maintain flexion.

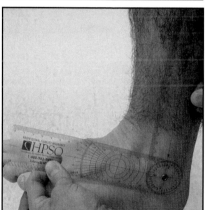

**Figure 4-24**. The ankle should be maximally dorsiflexed at the end of the movement.

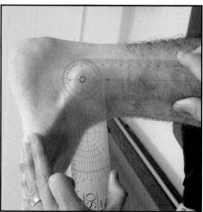

**Figure 4-25**. The patient may lie prone with the knee maintained in at least 30 degrees of flexion.

# Ankle Plantarflexion

**Planes/axis of movement:** Motion occurs in the sagittal plane around a coronal axis.

**Range of motion:**

- 0 degrees to 45 degrees

**Preferred starting position:** See Figure 4-26.

**End position:** See Figure 4-27.

**Goniometric alignment:**

- Axis: Center over the lateral aspect of the lateral malleolus
- Stationary arm: Align with the lateral midline of the fibula, siting the fibular head
- Moving arm: Align parallel to the lateral midline of the calcaneus

**Stabilization:** The tibia and fibula must be stabilized by the clinician (or on a supporting surface if the patient is in supine or prone) to prevent knee or hip motion.

**Substitutions:** The patient may try to extend the knee or hip to gain more range of motion during testing.

**Alternate method/position for testing:** See Figure 4-28.

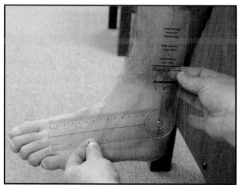

**Figure 4-26**. The patient is in sitting or supine with the knee flexed to at least 30 degrees. The foot should be in midposition between inversion and eversion. A towel roll is placed under the knee to maintain flexion.

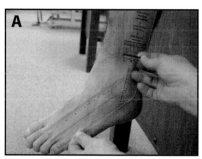
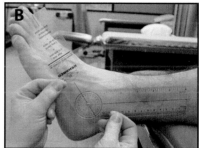

**Figure 4-27**. The ankle should be maximally plantarflexed at the end of the movement.

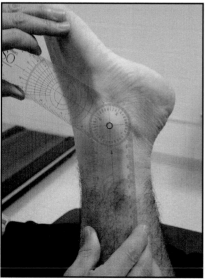

**Figure 4-28**. The patient may lie prone with the knee maintained in at least 30 degrees of flexion.

# THE SUBTALAR JOINT (HINDFOOT)

**Type of joint:** The subtalar joint is a complex joint in which the inferior surface of the talus articulates with the calcaneus, navicular, and cuboid bones. Movement occurs along an oblique axis allowing for foot inversion and eversion. This axis is located along a line that originates on the lateral posterior aspect of the heel and continues in an anterior-superior medial direction.

**Capsular pattern:** None.

## Subtalar Joint Inversion

**Planes/axis of movement:** This motion occurs in the frontal plane around an anterior/posterior axis in the anatomical position but occurs in the transverse plane around a vertical axis during testing.

**Range of motion:**

- 0 degrees to 30 degrees

**Preferred starting position:** See Figure 4-29.

**End position:** See Figure 4-30.

**Goniometric alignment:**

- Axis: Center over the posterior aspect of the ankle midway between the malleoli
- Stationary arm: Align with the posterior midline of the lower leg
- Moving arm: Align with the posterior midline of the calcaneus

**Stabilization:** The lower leg must be stabilized on a supporting surface to prevent hip or knee motion.

**Substitutions:** The patient may try to rotate the hip or flex the knee to increase motion during testing.

**Alternate method/position for testing:** None.

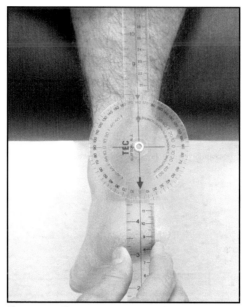

**Figure 4-29.** The patient is in prone with the hip in neutral position. The knee is in full extension with the foot over the edge of the supporting surface.

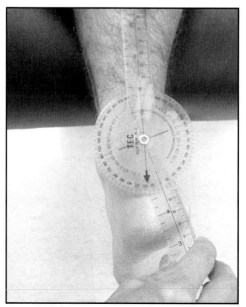

**Figure 4-30.** The hindfoot is in a position of maximal inversion at the end of the movement.

## Subtalar Eversion

**Planes/axis of movement:** This motion occurs in the frontal plane around an anterior/posterior axis in the anatomical position, but occurs in the transverse plane around a vertical axis during testing.

**Range of motion:**

- 0 degrees to 25 degrees

**Preferred starting position:** See Figure 4-31.

**End position:** See Figure 4-32.

**Goniometric alignment:**

- Axis: Center over the posterior aspect of the ankle midway between the malleoli

- Stationary arm: Align with the posterior midline of the lower leg

- Moving arm: Align with the posterior midline of the calcaneus

**Stabilization:** The lower leg must be stabilized on a supporting surface to prevent knee and hip movement.

**Substitutions:** The patient may try to rotate the hip or flex the knee to increase the range of motion during testing.

**Alternate method/position for testing:** None.

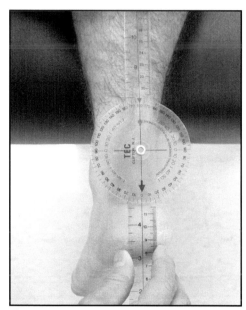

**Figure 4-31**. The patient is in prone with the hip in neutral position. The knee is in full extension with the foot over the edge of the supporting surface.

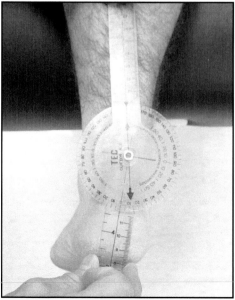

**Figure 4-32**. The hindfoot should be in a position of maximal eversion at the end of the movement.

# THE TRANSVERSE TARSAL (MIDTARSAL) JOINT

**Type of joint:** This is a complex joint that involves the articulations of the talus and calcaneus proximally and the navicular and cuboid distally. The calcaneocuboid joint is saddle shaped and the talonavicular joint acts in a similar manner to a hinged type of joint, with the convex surface of the talus articulating with the concave surface of the navicular. The movements of midfoot inversion and eversion occur at this joint.

There is also motion that exists between the midfoot and forefoot, which includes movements that occur at the tarsometatarsal joints. These are the articulations between the cuboid and 3 cuneiform bones with the bases of the 5 metatarsals. A slight amount of flexion and extension occurs with some rotary motion around the metatarsal joints, allowing the foot to move in an arc fashion.

**Capsular pattern:** None.

## Midtarsal Inversion

**Planes/axis of movement:** Movement is a combination of supination, adduction, and plantarflexion. The motion is measured in the frontal plane around an anterior/posterior axis because of the limitation of the goniometer to measure in a singular plane.

**Range of motion:**

- 0 degrees to 30 degrees

**Preferred starting position:** See Figure 4-33.

**End position:** See Figure 4-34.

**Goniometric alignment:**

- Axis: Center over the anterior aspect of the ankle midway between the malleoli

- Stationary arm: Align along the anterior midline of the tibial crest, siting the tibial tuberosity

- Moving arm: Align along the dorsal aspect of the second metatarsal shaft

**Stabilization:** The lower leg should be stabilized by the clinician (or on a supporting surface if the patient is in supine).

**Substitutions:** The patient may try to rotate the hip and knee to increase the range of motion during testing.

**Alternate method/position for testing:** See Figure 4-35.

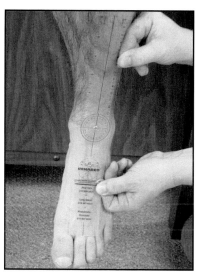

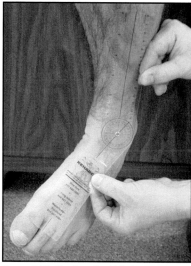

**Figure 4-33.** The patient sits with the knee flexed to 90 degrees.

**Figure 4-34.** The foot should be in a position of maximal inversion at the end of the movement.

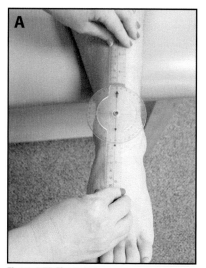

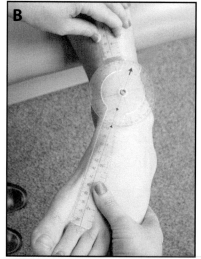

**Figure 4-35.** The patient may also be placed in supine with the hip and knee in extension and in neutral rotation. (A) Alternate starting position. (B) End position.

# Midtarsal Eversion

**Planes/axis of movement:** Movement is a combination of pronation, abduction, and dorsiflexion. Motion is measured in the frontal plane around an anterior/posterior axis because of the limitation of the goniometer to measure in a singular plane.

**Range of motion:**

- 0 degrees to 25 degrees

**Preferred starting position:** See Figure 4-36.

**End position:** See Figure 4-37.

**Goniometric alignment:**

- Axis: Center over the anterior aspect of the ankle midway between the malleoli

- Stationary arm: Align along the anterior midline of the tibial crest, siting the tibial tuberosity

- Moving arm: Align along the dorsal aspect of the second metatarsal shaft

**Stabilization:** The lower leg should be stabilized by the clinician (or on a supporting surface if the patient is in supine).

**Substitutions:** The patient may try to rotate the hip or knee to increase the range of motion during testing.

**Alternate method/position for testing:** See Figure 4-38.

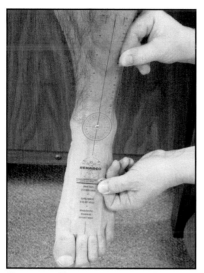

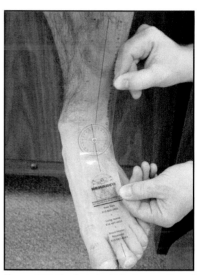

**Figure 4-36**. The patient is sitting with the knee flexed to 90 degrees.

**Figure 4-37**. The foot should be in a position of maximal eversion at the end of the movement.

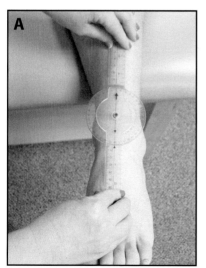

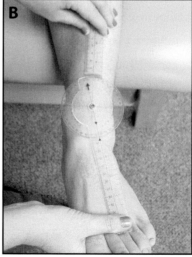

**Figure 4-38**. The patient may also be placed in supine with the hip and knee in extension and in neutral position. (A) Alternate starting position. (B) End position.

# THE FIRST TOE (METATARSOPHALANGEAL JOINT)

**Type of joint:** These joints are of the condyloid type and allow for 2 degrees of freedom, allowing for flexion/extension and abduction/adduction movements.

**Capsular pattern:** Great toe—extension > flexion.

## MTP Flexion

**Planes/axis of movement:** Motion occurs in the sagittal plane around a coronal axis.

**Range of motion:**

- 0 degrees to 45 degrees

**Preferred starting position:** See Figure 4-39.

**End position:** See Figure 4-40.

**Goniometric alignment:**

- Axis: Center over the dorsal aspect of the first metatarsophalangeal (MTP) joint
- Stationary arm: Align along the dorsal midline of the shaft of the first metatarsal
- Moving arm: Align along the dorsal midline of the proximal phalanx

**Stabilization:** The lower leg should be stabilized on a supporting surface and first metatarsal of the foot should be stabilized.

**Substitutions:** The patient may try to attempt to plantarflex the ankle to increase the range of motion during testing.

**Alternate method/position for testing:** None.

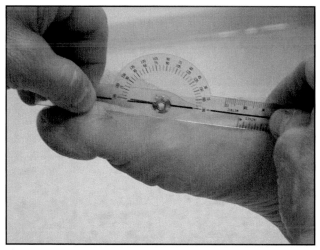

**Figure 4-39**. The patient may be in either sitting or supine with the ankle and foot in a neutral position over the edge of a table.

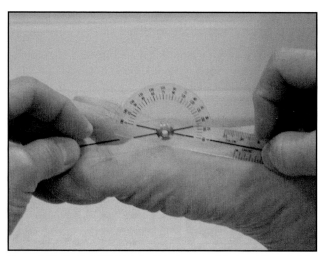

**Figure 4-40**. The first MTP joint should be in maximal flexion at the end of the movement.

GONIO

# MTP Extension/Hyperextension

**Planes/axis of movement:** Motion occurs in the sagittal plane around a coronal axis. Extension of the MTP joint is the return motion from MTP flexion.

**Range of motion:**

- 45 degrees to 0 degrees of extension
- 0 degrees to 90 degrees of hyperextension

**Preferred starting position:** See Figure 4-41.

**End position:** See Figure 4-42.

**Goniometric alignment:**

- Axis: Center over the dorsal aspect of the first MTP joint
- Stationary arm: Align along the dorsal midline of the shaft of the first metatarsal
- Moving arm: Align along the dorsal midline of the proximal phalanx

**Stabilization:** The lower leg should be stabilized on a supporting surface and the first metatarsal of the foot should be stabilized.

**Substitutions:** The patient may attempt to dorsiflex the ankle to increase the range of motion during testing.

**Alternate method/position for testing:** See Figure 4-43.

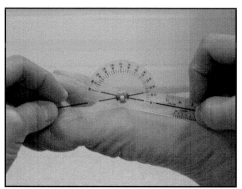

**Figure 4-41**. The patient may be in sitting or supine with the ankle and foot in neutral position over the edge of a table. The first MTP joint should be in full flexion.

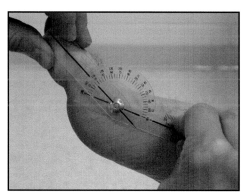

**Figure 4-42**. The first MTP joint should be in a position of maximal extension/ hyperextension at the end of the movement.

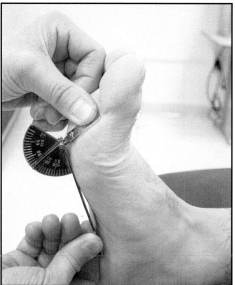

**Figure 4-43**. This motion may also be measured on the plantar surface of the first MTP joint.

# MTP Abduction

**Planes/axis of movement:** Motion occurs in the transverse plane around a vertical axis in the anatomical position.

**Range of motion:**

- The range of motion of the tested toe should be equal when compared to the nontested toe

**Preferred starting position:** See Figure 4-44.

**End position:** See Figure 4-45.

**Goniometric alignment:**

- Axis: Center over the dorsal aspect of the first MTP joint
- Stationary arm: Align with the dorsal midline of the first metatarsal
- Moving arm: Align with the dorsal midline of the proximal phalanx

**Stabilization:** The first metatarsal should be stabilized to prevent inversion or eversion of the foot.

**Substitutions:** The patient may try to invert the foot to avoid pain with motion.

**Alternate method/position for testing:** None.

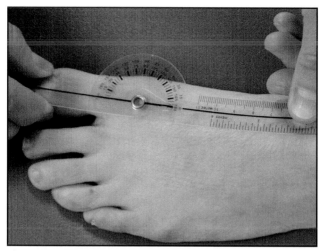

**Figure 4-44**. The patient should be placed in sitting or supine with the ankle and foot in neutral position between inversion and eversion. The MTP and interphalangeal (IP) joints should be in a neutral position between flexion and extension.

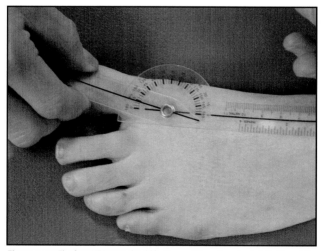

**Figure 4-45**. The first MTP joint should be in a position of maximal abduction at the end of the movement.

# THE FIRST TOE (INTERPHALANGEAL JOINT)

**Type of joint:** Hinge joint with 1 degree of freedom, allowing for flexion and extension only.

**Capsular pattern:** Flexion > extension.

## IP Flexion

**Planes/axis of movement:** Motion occurs in the sagittal plane around a coronal axis.

**Range of motion:**

- 0 degrees to 90 degrees

**Preferred starting position:** See Figure 4-46.

**End position:** See Figure 4-47.

**Goniometric alignment:**

- Axis: Align over the dorsal aspect of the IP joint
- Stationary arm: Align along the dorsal midline of the shaft of the proximal phalanx
- Moving arm: Align over the dorsal midline of the shaft of the distal phalanx

**Stabilization:** The lower leg should be stabilized on a supporting surface and the proximal phalanx should be stabilized.

**Substitutions:** The patient may try to plantarflex the ankle during testing to increase the range of motion.

**Alternate method/position for testing:** None.

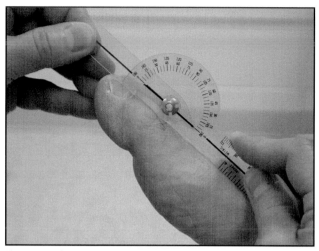

**Figure 4-46**. The patient should lie in supine with the foot/ankle in a neutral position over the edge of a table.

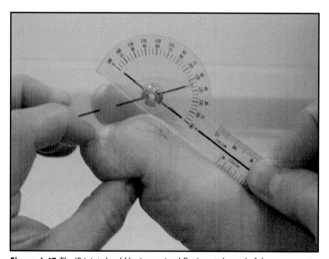

**Figure 4-47**. The IP joint should be in maximal flexion at the end of the movement.

# IP Extension/Hyperextension

**Planes/axis of movement:** Motion occurs in the sagittal plane around a coronal axis.

**Range of motion:**

- 90 degrees to 0 degrees; hyperextension is minimal

**Preferred starting position:** See Figure 4-48.

**End position:** See Figure 4-49.

**Goniometric alignment:**

- Axis: Align over the dorsal aspect of the IP joint

- Stationary arm: Align over the dorsal midline of the shaft of the proximal phalanx

- Moving arm: Align over the dorsal midline of the shaft of the distal phalanx

**Stabilization:** The lower leg should be stabilized on a supporting surface and the proximal phalanx should be stabilized.

**Substitutions:** The patient may try to dorsiflex the ankle during testing to gain more range of motion.

**Alternate method/position for testing:** See Figure 4-50.

GONIO

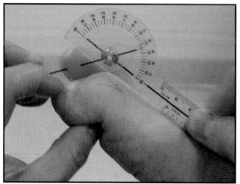

**Figure 4-48**. The patient should lie supine with the foot/ankle in a neutral position over the edge of a table. The IP joint should be in full flexion.

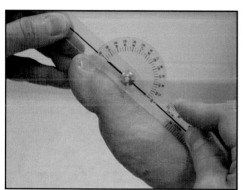

**Figure 4-49**. The IP joint should be in maximal extension/hyperextension at the end of the movement.

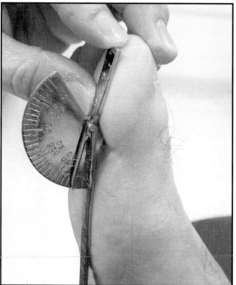

**Figure 4-50**. The goniometer may be placed on the plantar surface of the IP joint to measure hyperextension.

# TOES II TO V (METATARSOPHALANGEAL JOINTS)

**Type of joint:** Hinge joint with 1 degree of freedom, allowing for flexion and extension only.

**Capsular pattern:** Flexion > extension.

## MTP Flexion

**Planes/axis of movement:** Motion occurs in the sagittal plane around a coronal axis.

**Range of motion:**

- 0 degrees to 40 degrees

**Preferred starting position:** See Figure 4-51.

**End position:** See Figure 4-52.

**Goniometric alignment:**

- Axis: Center over the dorsal aspect of the tested MTP joint

- Stationary arm: Align over the dorsal midline of the metatarsal bone

- Moving arm: Align over the dorsal midline of the proximal phalanx

**Stabilization:** The metatarsals must be stabilized to prevent foot and ankle movement.

**Substitutions:** The patient may attempt to plantarflex the ankle to avoid pain with testing or increase the range of motion.

**Alternate method/position for testing:** None.

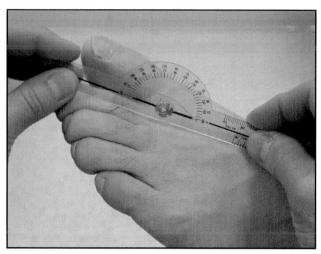

**Figure 4-51**. The patient should lie in supine with the foot/ankle in a neutral position over the edge of a table.

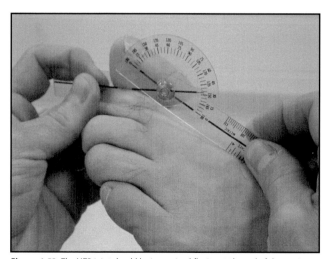

**Figure 4-52**. The MTP joint should be in maximal flexion at the end of the motion.

# MTP Extension/Hyperextension

**Planes/axis of movement:** This is the return motion from MTP flexion. Motion occurs in the sagittal plane around a coronal axis. The proximal phalanx glides dorsally on the metatarsal.

**Range of motion:**

- 40 degrees to 0 degrees (extension)
- 0 degrees to 45 (hyperextension)

**Preferred starting position:** See Figure 4-53.

**End position:** See Figure 4-54.

**Goniometric alignment:**

- Axis: Center over the dorsal aspect of the testing MTP joint
- Stationary arm: Align over the dorsal midline of the metatarsal bone
- Moving arm: Align over the dorsal midline of the proximal phalanx

**Stabilization:** The metatarsals must be stabilized to prevent foot and ankle movement.

**Substitutions:** The patient may attempt to dorsiflex the ankle to avoid pain with testing or increase the range of motion.

**Alternate method/position for testing:** See Figure 4-55.

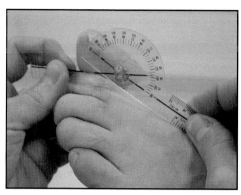

**Figure 4-53**. The patient lies supine with the foot/ankle in a neutral position over the edge of a table. The MTP joint should be in full flexion.

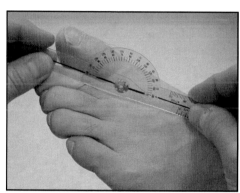

**Figure 4-54**. The MTP joint should be in a position of maximal extension at the end of the movement.

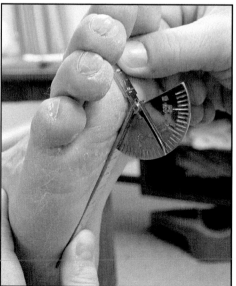

**Figure 4-55**. The goniometer may be placed on the plantar surface of the MTP joint to measure hyperextension.

# TOES II TO V (PROXIMAL INTERPHALANGEAL JOINTS)

**Type of joint:** These joints are hinge joints with 1 degree of freedom, allowing for flexion and extension only.

**Capsular pattern:** Flexion > extension.

## PIP Flexion

**Planes/axis of movement:** Motion occurs in the sagittal plane around a coronal axis.

**Range of motion:**

- 0 degrees to 35 degrees for toes II to V

**Preferred starting position:** See Figure 4-56.

**End position:** See Figure 4-57.

**Goniometric alignment:**

- Axis: Center over the dorsal aspect of the proximal interphalangeal (PIP) joint
- Stationary arm: Align along the dorsal midline of the shaft of the proximal phalanx
- Moving arm: Align along the dorsal midline of the shaft of the middle phalanx

**Stabilization:** The proximal phalanx and metatarsals of the foot should be stabilized.

**Substitutions:** The patient may try to plantarflex the ankle during testing to increase the range of motion.

**Alternate method/position for testing:** None.

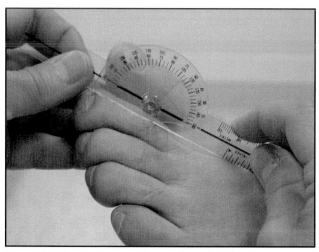

**Figure 4-56**. The patient may be sitting or supine with the foot/ankle in a neutral position over the edge of a table.

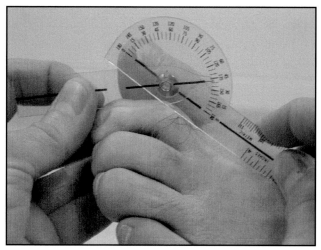

**Figure 4-57**. The PIP joint being tested should be in a position of maximal flexion at the end of the movement.

# PIP Extension

**Planes/axis of movement:** Motion occurs in the sagittal plane around a coronal axis.

**Range of motion:**

- 35 degrees to 0 degrees; hyperextension is minimal

**Preferred starting position:** See Figure 4-58.

**End position:** See Figure 4-59.

**Goniometric alignment:**

- Axis: Center over the dorsal aspect of the PIP joint

- Stationary arm: Align along the dorsal midline of the shaft of the proximal phalanx

- Moving arm: Align along the dorsal midline of the shaft of the middle phalanx

**Stabilization:** The proximal phalanx and metatarsals of the foot should be stabilized.

**Substitutions:** The patient may try to dorsiflex the ankle during testing in an attempt to increase the range of motion.

**Alternate method/position for testing:** None.

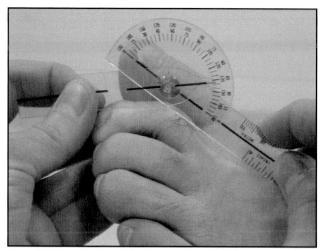

**Figure 4-58**. The patient may be in sitting or supine with the foot/ankle in a neutral position over the edge of a table. The PIP joint should be in full flexion.

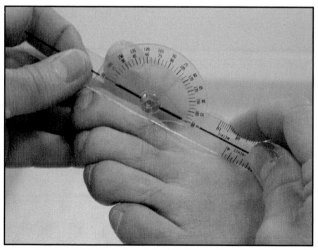

**Figure 4-59**. The PIP joint being tested should be in a position of maximal extension at the end of the movement.

# TOES II TO V (DISTAL INTERPHALANGEAL JOINTS)

**Type of joint:** These joints are hinge joints with 1 degree of freedom, allowing for flexion and extension only.

**Capsular pattern:** Flexion > extension.

## DIP Flexion

**Planes/axis of movement:** The motion occurs in the sagittal plane around a coronal axis.

**Range of motion:**

- 0 degrees to 60 degrees

**Preferred starting position:** See Figure 4-60.

**End position:** See Figure 4-61.

**Goniometric alignment:**

- Axis: Center over the dorsal aspect of the distal interphalangeal (DIP) joint
- Stationary arm: Align along the dorsal midline of the shaft of the middle phalanx
- Moving arm: Align along the dorsal midline of the shaft of the distal phalanx

**Stabilization:** The middle and proximal phalanges should be stabilized.

**Substitutions:** The patient may attempt to plantarflex the ankle or flex the MTP or PIP joints to increase the range of motion.

**Alternate method/position for testing:** None.

GONIO

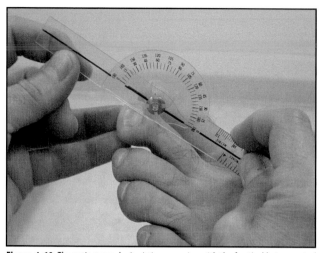

**Figure 4-60**. The patient may be in sitting or supine with the foot/ankle in a neutral position over the edge of a table.

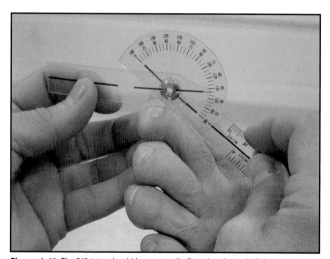

**Figure 4-61**. The DIP joint should be maximally flexed at the end of the movement.

# DIP Extension

**Planes/axis of movement:** Movement occurs in the sagittal plane around a coronal axis.

**Range of motion:**

- 60 degrees to 0 degrees; hyperextension is minimal

**Preferred starting position:** See Figure 4-62.

**End position:** See Figure 4-63.

**Goniometric alignment:**

- Axis: Center over the dorsal aspect of the DIP joint
- Stationary arm: Align over the dorsal midline of the middle phalanx
- Moving arm: Align over the dorsal midline of the distal phalanx

**Stabilization:** The middle and proximal phalanges should be stabilized.

**Substitutions:** The patient may attempt to dorsiflex the ankle or extend the MTP or PIP joints during testing to increase the range of motion.

**Alternate method/position for testing:** None.

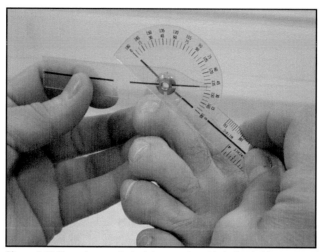

**Figure 4-62.** The patient may be in sitting or supine with the foot/ankle in a neutral position over the edge of a table. The DIP joint should be in full flexion.

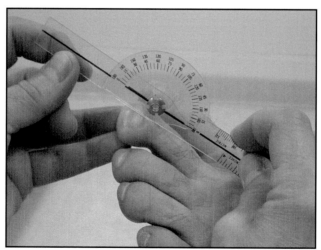

**Figure 4-63.** The DIP joint should be in a position of maximal extension at the end of the movement.

# THE TEMPOROMANDIBULAR JOINT

**Type of joint:** This is a complex joint that allows for opening, closing, protrusion, retrusion, and lateral deviation of the jaw. The temporomandibular joint is composed of the mandibular condyle and articulating surface of the glenoid fossa of the temporal bone. Between the mandibular condyle and glenoid fossa is an articulating disc or meniscus. During the opening of the jaw, a hinge type of motion is followed by a gliding motion of the condyle and the condyle moves down and out of the glenoid fossa on the disc. The disc then moves forward on the tubercle of the zygomatic process to complete the motion.

**Capsular pattern:** Restrictions in the ability to open the mouth.

## Depression of the Mandible (Opening of the Mouth)

**Planes/axis of movement:** Motion occurs in the sagittal plane around a coronal axis.

**Range of motion:**

- Approximately 2 inches or 3.5 to 4.0 cm; also equal to the width of 3 fingers between the teeth

**Preferred starting position:** The patient should be in sitting with the cervical spine in neutral.

**End position:** See Figure 5-1.

**Measurement of motion:** The movement is measured with a tape measure or ruler. The distance between the upper central incisor teeth and lower central incisor teeth is recorded.

**Stabilization:** The head and neck should be stabilized to prevent motion of the cervical spine during testing.

**Substitutions:** The patient may try to flex the cervical spine or retract the head to increase the range of motion or avoid pain during testing.

**Alternate method/position for testing:** None.

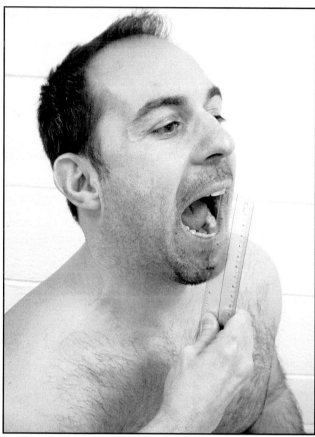

**Figure 5-1**. The patient should be sitting with the cervical spine in neutral. The mouth should be open as far as possible at end of the motion.

# Anterior Protrusion of the Mandible

**Planes/axis of movement:** Motion occurs in the transverse plane and is a translatory type of motion.

**Range of motion:**

- Normal motion is the ability of the lower central incisor teeth to move forward beyond the upper central incisor teeth

**Preferred starting position:** The patient should be in sitting with the cervical spine in a neutral position.

**End position:** See Figure 5-2.

**Measurement of motion:** The movement is measured with a tape measure or ruler. The distance between the lower central incisor teeth and upper central incisor teeth is measured.

**Stabilization:** The head and neck should be stabilized to prevent motion of the cervical spine during testing.

**Substitutions:** The patient may attempt to extend the cervical spine or protrude the head to avoid pain or increase the range of motion during testing.

**Alternate method/position for testing:** None.

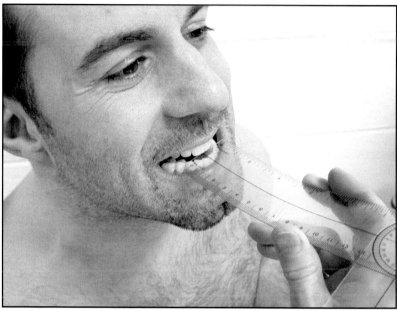

**Figure 5-2.** The patient should be sitting with the cervical spine in a neutral position. The mandible should be protruded as far as possible at the end of the movement.

## Lateral Protrusion of the Mandible

**Planes/axis of movement:** Motion occurs in the transverse plane and is a translatory type of motion.

**Range of motion:**

- Normal amount of motion allows for a comparable amount of lateral motion to both the right and left sides

**Preferred starting position:** The patient should be in sitting with the cervical spine in a neutral position.

**End position:** See Figure 5-3.

**Measurement of motion:** The movement is measured with a tape measure or ruler. The distance between the most lateral points of the lower and upper cuspid teeth or first bicuspid teeth are recorded.

**Stabilization:** The head and neck should be stabilized to prevent motion of the cervical spine during testing.

**Substitutions:** The patient may try to rotate the cervical spine to avoid pain or increase the range of motion during testing.

**Alternate method/position for testing:** None.

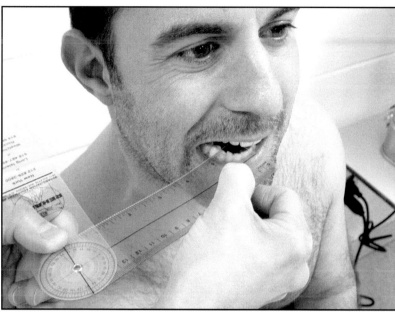

**Figure 5-3**. The patient should be sitting with cervical spine in a neutral position. The mandible should be in a position of maximal lateral protrusion at the end of the movement.

# MANUAL MUSCLE TESTING

# Key to Manual Muscle Grading

| | Muscle Activity | Kendall | | | Daniels & Worthingham | |
|---|---|---|---|---|---|---|
| No movement | No contraction felt in muscle | 0 | 0 | Zero | 0 | Zero |
| | Tendon is prominent and muscle contraction is palpable, no visible movement of tested body part | Trace | 1 | Trace | 1 | Trace |
| | *Gravity Minimized Position* | | | | | |
| Test movement | Moves through partial range of motion | 1 | 2– | Poor– | 2– | Poor– |
| | Moves through complete range of motion | 2 | 2 | Poor | 2 | Poor |
| | *Anti-Gravity Position* | | | | | |
| Test position | Moves through partial range of motion | 3 | 2+ | Poor+ | 2+ | Poor+ |
| | Gradual release from test position | 4 | 3– | Fair– | | |
| | Holds test position with no resistance | 5 | 3 | Fair | 3 | Fair |
| | Holds test position against slight resistance | 6 | 3+ | Fair+ | 3+ | Fair+ |
| | Holds test position against slight to moderate resistance | 7 | 4– | Good– | | |
| | Holds test position against moderate resistance | 8 | 4 | Good | 4 | Good |
| | Holds test position against moderate to strong resistance | 9 | 4+ | Good+ | | |
| | Holds test position against strong resistance | 10 | 5 | Normal | 5 | Normal |

MMT

# SECTION VI

# Neck/Upper Extremities

# NECK

## Flexion

### Active Range of Motion

- 0 degrees to 45 degrees with a goniometer
- 1.0 cm to 4.3 cm with a tape measure

### Prime Movers

- Sternocleidomastoid
    - ☐ Origin
        - o Sternal head: Cranial aspect of the ventral surface of the manubrium
        - o Clavicular head: Superior border and anterior surface of the medial one-third of the clavicle
    - ☐ Insertion: Lateral surface of the mastoid process and lateral half of the superior nuchal line of the occipital bone
    - ☐ Innervation: Spinal accessory nerve (C2 and C3 anterior rami)
    - ☐ Other actions: Lateral flexion (to the same side) and rotation (to the opposite side) of the neck/head
    - ☐ Palpation site: Anterolateral aspect of the neck

### Secondary Movers

- Rectus capitits anterior
- Rectus capitis lateralis
- Suprahyoid
- Infrahyoid
- Platysma
- Scalenes
- Longus capitis
- Longus colli

## Anti-Gravity

**Patient position:** Supine on a table.

**Stabilization:** Weight of the trunk and clinician's hand on the thorax.

- Grades 5/5 to +3/5: See Figure 6-1

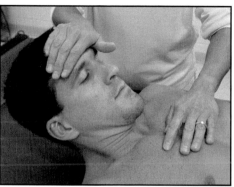

**Figure 6-1.** Resistance is applied to the anterior forehead.

PATIENT DIRECTIVE: *"Lift your head up off the table. Do not lift your shoulders up and do not let me push your head down."*

*\*The 2 sternocleidomastoid muscles may be tested individually by rotation of the head to one side with neck flexion.*

- Grade 3/5: See Figure 6-2

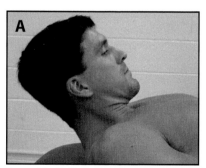
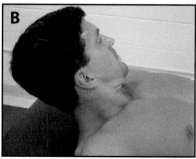

**Figure 6-2.** (A) The patient flexes the neck through the maximal range of motion without resistance. (B) Cervical rotation with flexion.

- Grades −3/5 to +2/5: See Figure 6-3

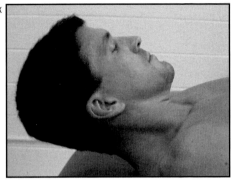

**Figure 6-3**. The patient flexes the neck through partial range of motion.

## Gravity Minimized

**Patient position:** Sidelying with the head supported on a smooth surface.

**Stabilization:** The clinician stabilizes the lower thorax.

- Grades 2/5 to −2/5: See Figure 6-4A
- Grade 2/5: See Figure 6-4B

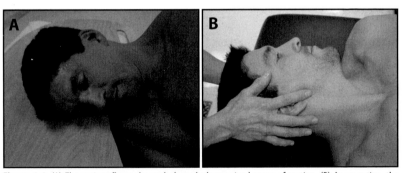

**Figure 6-4**. (A) The patient flexes the neck through the maximal range of motion. (B) As an option, the patient may be asked to rotate the head to 1 side and then to the other.

- Grades 1/5 to 0/5: See Figure 6-5

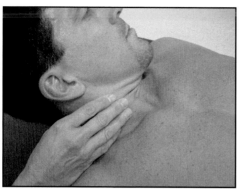

**Figure 6-5.** The sternocleidomastoid muscles are palpated on the sides of the neck while the patient attempts to flex.

**Substitutions:** The corners of the patient's mouth may be pulled down if the platysma contracts.

**Points of interest:** Torticollis may result if the sternocleidomastoid becomes dystonic.

# Extension

## Active Range of Motion

- 0 degrees to 45 degrees

## Prime Movers

- Splenius capitis
  - ☐ Origin: Caudal half of the ligamentum nuchae and spinous processes of C7 and T1 to T4 vertebrae
  - ☐ Insertion: Occipital bone just inferior to the lateral one-third of the superior nuchal line into the mastoid process of the temporal bone
  - ☐ Innervation: Lateral branches of the dorsal primary cervical nerves
  - ☐ Other actions: Slight rotation and lateral flexion of the head
  - ☐ Palpation site: Under the lateral borders of the upper trapezius

- Semispinalis capitis
  - ☐ Origin: Tips of the transverse processes of the C7 and T1 to T7 vertebrae
  - ☐ Insertion: Between the superior and inferior nuchal lines of the occipital bone
  - ☐ Innervation: Dorsal primary divisions of the cervical nerves
  - ☐ Other actions: Unilaterally: Rotation of the spine to the opposite side
  - ☐ Palpation site: Under the lateral borders of the upper trapezius

- Cervicis muscles
  - ☐ Origin: Spinous processes of the T3 to T6 vertebrae
  - ☐ Insertion: Posterior tubercles of C1 to C3
  - ☐ Innervation: Dorsal primary branch of the spinal nerves
  - ☐ Other actions: Unilaterally: Lateral flexion and rotation of the head
  - ☐ Palpation site: Under the lateral borders of the upper trapezius

## Secondary Movers

- Upper trapezius

## Anti-Gravity

**Patient position:** Prone on a table.

**Stabilization:** Weight of the trunk and the clinician's hand on the upper thoracic area and scapulae.

- Grades 5/5 to +3/5: See Figure 6-6

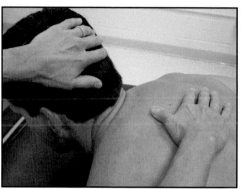

**Figure 6-6.** Resistance is applied to the occiput.

PATIENT DIRECTIVE: *"Lift your head up toward the ceiling. Do not let me push your head down."*

- Grade 3/5: See Figure 6-7

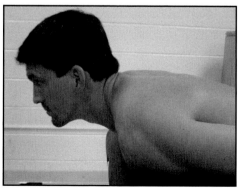

**Figure 6-7.** The patient extends the neck through the maximal range of motion without resistance.

MMT

- Grades −3/5 to +2/5: See Figure 6-8

**Figure 6-8**. The patient extends the neck through partial range of motion.

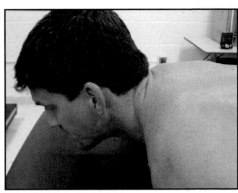

## Gravity Minimized

**Patient position:** Sidelying with the head supported on a smooth surface.

**Stabilization:** Weight of the trunk on the table.

- Grades 2/5 to −2/5: See Figure 6-9

**Figure 6-9**. The patient extends the neck through the maximal range of motion.

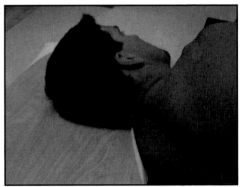

- Grades 1/5 to 0/5: See Figure 6-10

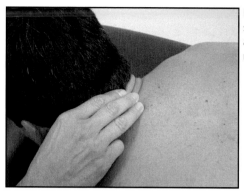

**Figure 6-10.** The splenius capitis, semispinalis capitis, and cervicis muscles are palpated on the posterior aspect of the neck while the patient tries to extend.

**Substitutions:** The patient may try to use the back muscles to lift the upper trunk from the table.

**Points of interest:** Tasks such as reaching overhead into a high cabinet, the top shelf in a closet, or drinking out of a cup require the contraction of the the cervical extensors at the end of the range of motion.

MMT

# SCAPULA

## Abduction/Upward Rotation

### Active Range of Motion

- Right and left sides should be symmetrical when measured with a tape measure

### Prime Movers

- Serratus anterior

  □ Origin: Anterior surfaces of ribs 1 through 9

  □ Insertion: Anterior aspect of the medial border of the scapula from superior to inferior angle

  □ Innervation: Long thoracic nerve (C5 to C7)

  □ Other actions: Stabilizes the scapula against the chest wall

  □ Palpation site: Along the midaxillary line adjacent to the inferior angle of the scapula

### Secondary Movers

- Pectoralis minor

### Anti-Gravity

**Patient position:** Supine with the shoulder flexed to 90 degrees and the elbow in extension.

**Stabilization:** Weight of the trunk against the table.

MMT

- Grades 5/5 to +3/5: See Figure 6-11

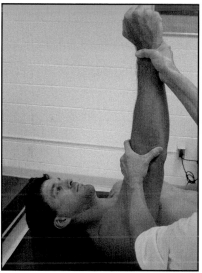

**Figure 6-11**. Resistance is given in a downward/inward direction by grasping the forearm and elbow.

PATIENT DIRECTIVE: *"Punch up toward the ceiling and resist as I push down."*

- Grades 3/5 to + 2/5: See Figure 6-12

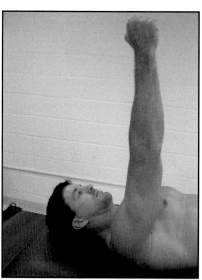

**Figure 6-12**. The patient moves the arm upward from a resting position on the table without resistance.

MMT

## Gravity Minimized

**Patient position:** Sitting with the upper arm resting on a table in 90 degrees of shoulder flexion and with the elbow extended.

**Stabilization:** Clinician stabilizes the thorax to prevent rotation or forward movement.

- Grades 2/5 to –2/5: See Figure 6-13

**Figure 6-13.** The patient moves the arm forward 2 to 3 inches by abducting the scapula through the maximal range of motion.

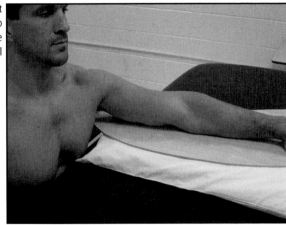

- Grades 1/5 to 0/5: See Figure 6-14

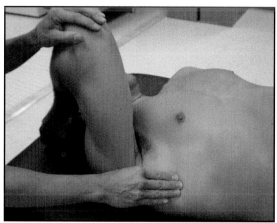

**Figure 6-14.** The serratus anterior is palpated along the midaxillary line adjacent to the inferior angle of the scapula as the patient attempts to abduct the scapula against light resistance.

**Points of interest:** Weakness of the serratus anterior causes "winging" of the scapula, which is most evident when standing and pushing against a wall. It is the strongest abductor of the scapula and weakness of this muscle makes it difficult to flex or abduct the shoulder.

MMT

## Adduction/Downward Rotation

### Active Range of Motion

- Right and left sides should be symmetrical when measured with a tape measure

### Prime Movers

- Rhomboid major

  □ Origin: Spinous processes of T2 to T5

  □ Insertion: Medial border of the scapula between the spine and inferior angle

  □ Innervation: Dorsal scapular nerve (C5)

  □ Other actions: Scapular stabilization

  □ Palpation site: With the patient's hand behind their lumbar spine, palpate under and along the medial border of the scapula

- Rhomboid minor

  □ Origin: Spinous processes of C7 and T1

  □ Insertion: The medial border of the scapula at the level of the spine of the scapula

  □ Innervation: Dorsal scapular nerve (C5)

  □ Other actions: Scapular stabilization

  □ Palpation site: With the patient's hand behind their lumbar spine, palpate under and along the medial border of the scapula

### Secondary Movers

- Middle trapezius

- Levator scapulae

### Anti-Gravity

**Patient position:** Prone with the tested upper extremity behind the back with the hand resting on the lumbar spine. The head is rotated to the opposite side.

**Stabilization:** The clinician stabilizes the thorax on the opposite side.

MMT

- Grades 5/5 to +3/5: See Figure 6-15

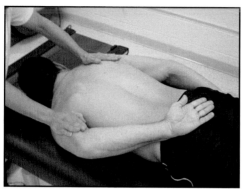

**Figure 6-15.** As the patient lifts their hand off the back, resistance is applied above the elbow in a down and out direction, pushing the scapula into abduction and upward rotation.

PATIENT DIRECTIVE: *"Lift your hand up toward the ceiling and do not let me push your arm down."*

- Grade 3/5: See Figure 6-16

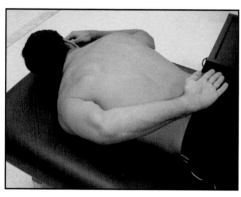

**Figure 6-16.** The patient lifts their hand off the back as the scapula is adducted through the maximal range of motion.

## Gravity Minimized

**Patient position:** Sitting with the tested arm internally rotated and adducted behind the lumbar spine.

**Stabilization:** The clinician stabilizes the anterior/posterior trunk if necessary to prevent flexion or rotation.

MMT

- Grades 2/5 to −2/5: See Figure 6-17

**Figure 6-17**. The patient attempts to adduct the scapula through the range of motion.

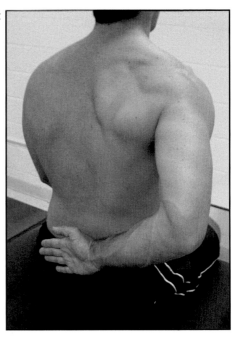

- Grades 1/5 to 0/5: See Figure 6-18

**Figure 6-18**. The rhomboids may be palpated under and along the medial border of the scapula as the patient attempts to adduct the scapula.

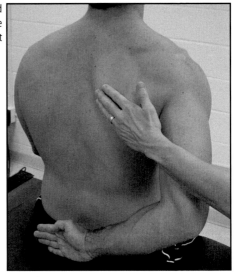

MMT

**Substitutions:** The latissimus dorsi and teres major may cause the shoulder to adduct and extend the shoulder without scapular rotation. The patient may use the wrist extensors to lift the upper extremity off the lower back without scapular movement.

**Points of interest:** Weakness of the rhomboids may cause medial scapular winging and decreased strength of shoulder adduction and extension due to loss of scapular stabilization.

MMT

# Elevation

## Prime Movers

- Upper trapezius

    □ Origin: External occipital protuberance, medial third superior nuchal line, and the ligamentum nuchae

    □ Insertion: Posterior border of the lateral third of the clavicle and acromion process

    □ Innervation: Spinal accessory nerve (CN XI)

    □ Other actions: Lateral rotation of the scapula

    □ Palpation site: The superior and posterior surface of the shoulders

- Levator scapulae

    □ Origin: Transverse processes of C1 to C4

    □ Insertion: Medial border of the scapula at the level of the scapular superior angle

    □ Innervation: Dorsal scapular nerve (C5) and C3, C4

    □ Other actions: Medial rotation of the scapula and scapular stabilization

    □ Palpation site: Deep to the upper trapezius in the angle formed by the upper trapezius and sternocleidomastoid muscles

## Secondary Movers

- Rhomboids major and minor

## Anti-Gravity

**Patient position:** Sitting in a chair or on a table with the arms hanging by the sides.

**Stabilization:** Achieved through patient compliance.

MMT

• Grades 5/5 to +3/5: See Figure 6-19

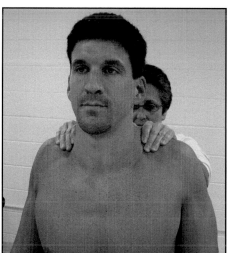

**Figure 6-19**. Resistance is applied symmetrically in a downward direction on top of the shoulders.

PATIENT DIRECTIVE: *"Raise your shoulders as high as possible toward the ceiling and hold while I try to push them down."*

• Grades 3/5 to +2/5: See Figure 6-20

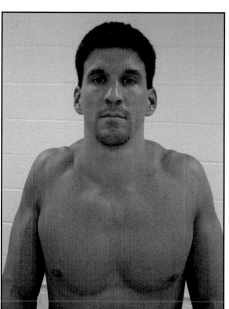

**Figure 6-20**. The patient elevates the shoulders through the maximal range of motion without resistance.

## Gravity Minimized

**Patient position:** Supine or prone on a table with the arms by the sides.

**Stabilization:** Weight of the trunk on the table.

- Grades 2/5 to –2/5: See Figure 6-21

**Figure 6-21**. As the clinician supports the shoulders, the patient elevates the shoulders toward the ears.

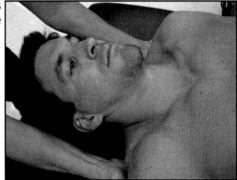

- Grades 1/5 to 0/5: See Figure 6-22

**Figure 6-22**. The upper trapezius is palpated to the cervical vertebrae and its insertion at the superior/posterior aspect of the distal clavicle as the patient attempts to elevate the shoulders.

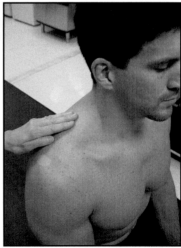

**Points of interest:** Weakness of the upper trapezius may cause lateral winging of the scapula, which is most obvious when attempting to abduct the shoulder. Weakness of the upper trapezius also causes difficulty when trying to abduct or flex the upper extremity above shoulder height.

## Adduction

### Active Range of Motion

- Right and left sides should be symmetrical when measured with a tape measure

### Prime Movers

- Middle trapezius

    □ Origin: Inferior aspect of the ligamentum nuchae, spinous processes of C7 to T5

    □ Insertion: Medial aspect of the acromion process and superior lip of the spine of the scapula

    □ Innervation: Spinal accessory nerve (CN XI)

    □ Other actions: None

    □ Palpation site: Medial border of the scapula near the root of the spine

- Rhomboid major

    □ Origin: Spinous processes of T2 to T5

    □ Insertion: Medial border of the scapula between the spine and inferior angle

    □ Innervation: Dorsal scapular nerve (C5)

    □ Other actions: Scapular stabilization

    □ Palpation site: With the patient's hand behind their lumbar spine, palpate under and along the medial border of the scapula

- Rhomboid minor

    □ Origin: Spinous processes of C7 to T1

    □ Insertion: The medial border of the scapula at the level of the spine of the scapula

    □ Innervation: Dorsal scapular nerve (C5)

    □ Other actions: Scapular stabilization

    □ Palpation site: With the patient's hand behind their lumbar spine, palpate under and along the medial border of the scapula

## Secondary Movers

- Upper and lower trapezius

## Anti-Gravity

**Patient position:** Prone on a table with the shoulder in 90 degrees of abduction and with the elbow flexed to 90 degrees, the forearm hanging freely over the edge of a table.

**Stabilization:** Weight of the trunk on the table. The clinician stabilizes the contralateral thorax.

- Grades 5/5 to +3/5: See Figure 6-23

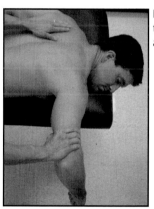

**Figure 6-23.** Resistance is applied just proximal to the elbow toward the floor as the patient horizontally abducts the shoulder and adducts the scapula.

PATIENT DIRECTIVE: *"Squeeze your shoulder blades together and push your arm up into my hand and hold it. Do not let me push your arm down."*

- Grades 3/5 to +2/5: See Figure 6-24

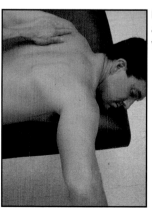

**Figure 6-24.** The patient raises their arm toward the ceiling while adducting the scapula through the available range of motion without resistance.

MMT

## Gravity Minimized

**Patient position:** Sitting with the arm resting on a table with the shoulder abducted to 90 degrees and the elbow flexed to 90 degrees.

**Stabilization:** The clinician stabilizes the contralateral thorax.

- Grades 2/5 to –2/5: See Figure 6-25

**Figure 6-25.** The patient horizontally abducts the shoulder and adducts the scapula through the available range of motion.

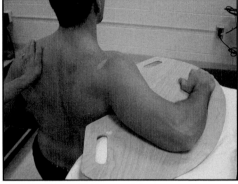

• Grades 1/5 to 0/5: See Figure 6-26

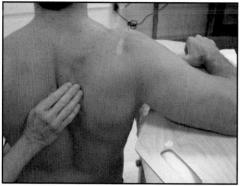

**Figure 6-26**. The middle trapezius is palpated along the medial border of the scapula between thoracaic vertebrae T1 to T5 and near the root of the spine of the scapula as the patient attempts to horizontally abduct the shoulder.

**Substitutions:** The posterior deltoid may cause horizontal abduction of the shoulder without scapular adduction. The lower trapezius may cause depression to occur and the rhomboids may slightly elevate and downwardly rotate the scapula.

MMT

## Depression/Adduction

### Prime Movers

- Lower trapezius

  - ☐ Origin: Spinous processes of T6 to T12

  - ☐ Insertion: The root and inferiorly on the spine of the scapula

  - ☐ Innervation: Spinal accessory nerve (CN XI)

  - ☐ Other actions: None

  - ☐ Palpation site: Medial to the root of the spine and the medial border of the scapula

### Secondary Movers

- Middle trapezius

- Pectoralis minor

- Latissimus dorsi

- Pectoralis major

- Pectoralis minor

### Anti-Gravity

**Patient position:** Prone with the head rotated to the same side and tested shoulder in approximately 130 degrees of abduction and with the elbow in extension.

**Stabilization:** The clinician stabilizes the contralateral thorax.

- Grades 5/5 to +3/5: See Figure 6-27

**Figure 6-27.** Resistance is applied just proximal to the elbow joint directed down toward the floor.

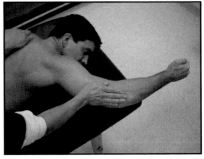

PATIENT DIRECTIVE: *"Raise your arm up off the table as far as you can and hold it. Do not let me push it down."*

- Grade 3/5: See Figure 6-28

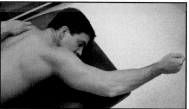

**Figure 6-28.** The patient lifts the limb off the table without resistance.

PATIENT DIRECTIVE: *"Raise your arm up off the table as far as you can and hold it. Do not let me push it down."*

*\*The upper extremity may be supported by the clinician into abduction if the deltoid is weak.*

## Gravity Minimized

**Patient position:** Prone with the head rotated to the same side as the tested shoulder in approximately 130 degrees of abduction.

**Stabilization:** The clinician stabilizes the contralateral thorax.

- Grade 2/5: See Figure 6-29

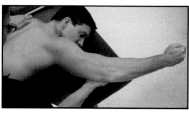

**Figure 6-29.** The patient is able to achieve full scapular movement with the tested limb supported.

- Grades 1/5 to 0/5: See Figure 6-30

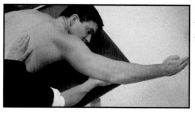

**Figure 6-30.** The lower trapezius is palpated medial to the root of the spine and medial border of the scapula as the patient attempts to lift the arm off the table.

MMT

**Substitutions:** The patient may try to extend the trunk to give the appearance of scapular movement.

# SHOULDER

## Flexion

### Active Range of Motion

- 0 degrees to 180 degrees

### Prime Movers

- Anterior deltoid
  - ☐ Origin: Anterior and superior lateral third of the clavicle
  - ☐ Insertion: Deltoid tuberosity of the humerus
  - ☐ Innervation: Axillary nerve (C5 to C6)
  - ☐ Other actions: Internally rotates and horizontally adducts the shoulder
  - ☐ Palpation site: Inferior to the lateral third of the clavicle
- Coracobrachialis (up to 90 degrees of shoulder flexion)
  - ☐ Origin: Coracoid process of the scapula
  - ☐ Insertion: Medial surface of the midshaft of the humerus
  - ☐ Innervation: Musculocutaneous nerve (C6 to C7)
  - ☐ Other actions: Scaption of the shoulder
  - ☐ Palpation site: Deep into the upper middle third of the arm, in the axilla, under the inferior border of the pectoralis major muscle

### Secondary Movers

- Middle deltoid
- Pectoralis major
- Biceps brachii

### Anti-Gravity

**Patient position:** Sitting with the shoulder flexed to 90 degrees, palm facing down.

**Stabilization:** The clinician stabilizes the opposite scapula.

MMT

- Grades 5/5 to +3/5: See Figure 6-31

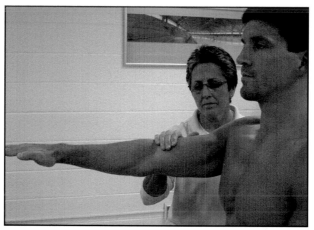

**Figure 6-31.** Resistance is applied in a downward direction just proximal to the elbow joint.

PATIENT DIRECTIVE: *"Hold your arm up and do not let me push it down."*

- Grades 3/5: See Figure 6-32

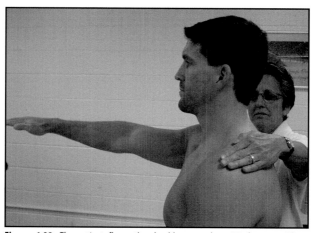

**Figure 6-32.** The patient flexes the shoulder to at least 90 degrees without resistance.

MMT

## Gravity Minimized

**Patient position:** Sidelying with the upper extremity supported on a smooth surface and in neutral rotation with the elbow in flexion.

**Stabilization:** The opposite shoulder is stabilized by the weight of the body against the table.

• Grades 2/5 to –2/5: See Figure 6-33

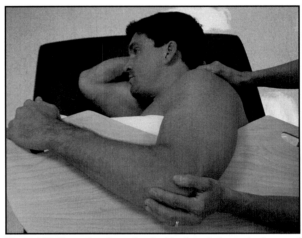

**Figure 6-33**. The patient flexes the shoulder through the maximal range of motion.

- Grades 1/5 to 0/5: See Figure 6-34

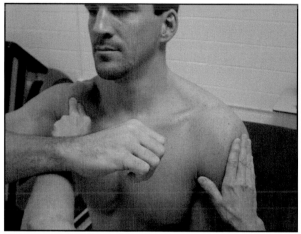

**Figure 6-34**. The anterior deltoid is palpated inferiorly to the lateral third of the clavicle. The coracobrachialis is palpated in the axilla along the inferior border of the pectoralis major muscle. (Shown: Palpating the anterior deltoid.)

**Substitutions:** If the upper trapezius is activated, the scapula will elevate. Substitution by the pectoralis major will cause horizontal adduction. The patient may also externally rotate the shoulder to substitute with the biceps or lean back into trunk extension to give the appearance of shoulder flexion.

MMT

# Extension

## Active Range of Motion

- 180 degrees to 0 degrees
- 0 degrees to 40/60 degrees (from neutral)

## Prime Movers

- Latissimus dorsi

    □ Origin: Lumbar aponeurosis, spinous processes of T6 to T12, L1 to L5, and the sacral vertebrae

    □ Insertion: Medial lip of the intertubercular groove of the humerus

    □ Innervation: Thoracodorsal nerve (C6 to C8)

    □ Other actions: Adducts and internally rotates the shoulder and assists with scapular depression

    □ Palpation site: Along the midaxillary line on the trunk

- Teres major

    □ Origin: Posterior surface of the inferior scapular angle

    □ Insertion: Crest of the lessor tubercle of the humerus

    □ Innervation: Lower subscapular nerve (C6)

    □ Other actions: Adduction and internal rotation of the shoulder

    □ Palpation site: Lateral to the inferior angle of the scapula

- Posterior deltoid

    □ Origin: Inferior lip of the posterior border of the spine of the scapula

    □ Insertion: Deltoid tuberosity of the humerus

    □ Innervation: Axillary nerve (C5 to C6)

    □ Other actions: External rotation and horizontal abduction of the shoulder

    □ Palpation site: Inferior and lateral to the spine of the scapula

## Secondary Movers

- Long head of the triceps brachii

## Anti-Gravity

**Patient position:** The patient should be prone with the arms at the sides and with the palm facing up toward the ceiling.

**Stabilization:** The weight of the thorax against the table.

- Grades 5/5 to +3/5: See Figure 6-35

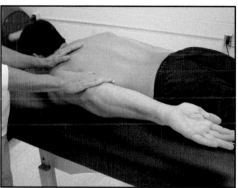

**Figure 6-35**. Resistance is applied at the elbow in a downward direction toward the floor.

PATIENT DIRECTIVE: *"Lift your arm as high as you can toward the ceiling and hold it. Do not let me push it down."*

- Grade 3/5: See Figure 6-36

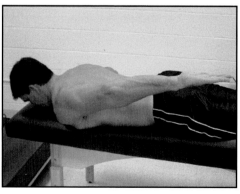

**Figure 6-36**. The patient lifts the arm up toward the ceiling through the maximal range of motion without resistance.

MMT

## Gravity Minimized

**Patient position:** Sidelying with the upper extremity supported on a smooth surface and in neutral rotation with the elbow in flexion.

**Stabilization:** The opposite shoulder is stabilized by the weight of the body against the table.

- Grades 2/5 to –2/5: See Figure 6-37

**Figure 6-37.** The patient extends the shoulder through the maximal range of motion.

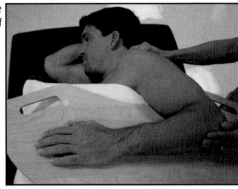

- Grades 1/5 to 0/5: See Figure 6-38

**Figure 6-38.** The latissimus dorsi is palpated inferiorly and lateral to the inferior angle of the scapula on the side of the thoracic wall as the patient attempts to extend the shoulder. The teres major and posterior deltoid are palpable at the lateral border of the scapula just below the axilla and just superior to the axilla, respectively. (Shown: Palpating the latissimus dorsi.)

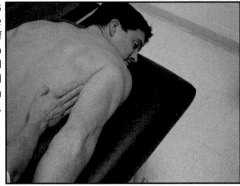

**Substitutions:** The patient may attempt to lift and rotate the trunk.

**Points of interest:** The latissimus dorsi is a powerful shoulder extensor and is active during forceful activities, such as swimming, rowing/paddling, or chopping movements. It pulls the shoulder girdle down during any activity that requires the body to be pulled toward the arm as in crutch walking or rock climbing. The teres major is occasionally known as the "little latissimus" because it performs the same actions as the latissimus dorsi. In combination with the infraspinatus and teres minor, it pulls downward to help stabilize the head of the humerus during abduction.

MMT

## Abduction

### Active Range of Motion

- 0 degrees to 180 degrees

### Prime Movers

- Middle deltoid

  ☐ Origin: Superior/lateral surface of the acromion process of the scapula

  ☐ Insertion: Deltoid tuberosity of the humerus

  ☐ Innervation: Axillary nerve (C5 to C6)

  ☐ Other actions: Scaption

  ☐ Palpation site: Lateral/inferior to the acromion process

### Secondary Movers

- Supraspinatus

### Anti-Gravity

**Patient position:** Sitting with the shoulder abducted to 90 degrees, palm down.

**Stabilization:** The clinician stabilizes the opposite shoulder.

- Grades 5/5 to +3/5: See Figure 6-39

**Figure 6-39.** Resistance is applied just proximal to the elbow in a downward direction toward the floor.

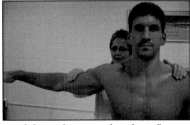

PATIENT DIRECTIVE: *"Hold your arm up and do not let me push it down."*

MMT

- Grade 3/5: See Figure 6-40

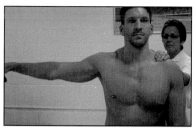

**Figure 6-40**. The patient abducts the shoulder to at least 90 degrees without resistance.

## Gravity Minimized

**Patient position:** Supine with the tested limb supported on a table.

**Stabilization:** Weight of the trunk on the table.

- Grades 2/5 to –2/5: See Figure 6-41

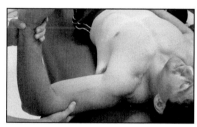

**Figure 6-41**. The patient abducts the shoulder through the maximal range of motion.

- Grades 1/5 to 0/5: See Figure 6-42

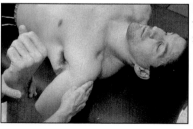

**Figure 6-42**. The middle deltoid is palpated lateral to the acrominon process on the superior aspect of the shoulder as the patient attempts to abduct the shoulder.

**Substitutions:** The patient may try to elevate the shoulder or laterally flex the trunk to give the illusion of shoulder abduction.

**Points of interest:** Although the deltoid is a strong abductor, it is the supraspinatus, not the deltoid, that initiates the movement because the angle of the pull of the middle deltoid is parallel to the shaft of the humerus when the upper extremity is positioned at the side.

MMT

## Horizontal Abduction

### Active Range of Motion

- 0 degrees to 45 degrees (from neutral)

### Prime Movers

- Posterior deltoid
    - ☐ Origin: Inferior lip of the posterior border of the spine of the scapula
    - ☐ Insertion: Deltoid tuberosity of the humerus
    - ☐ Innervation: Axillary nerve (C5 to C6)
    - ☐ Other actions: Extends and externally rotates the shoulder
    - ☐ Palpation site: Inferior/lateral to the spine of the scapula

### Secondary Movers

- Long head of the triceps brachii

### Anti-Gravity

**Patient position:** Prone with the shoulder in 90 degrees of abduction and with the forearm off the edge of the table with the elbow in flexion.

**Stabilization:** Weight of the trunk on the table.

- Grades 5/5 to +3/5: See Figure 6-43

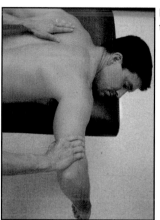

**Figure 6-43**. Resistance is applied just proximal to the elbow toward the floor.

PATIENT DIRECTIVE: *"Lift your elbow up toward the ceiling and hold it. Do not let me push it down."*

- Grades 3/5 to +2/5: See Figure 6-44

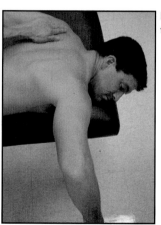

**Figure 6-44**. The patient horizontally abducts the shoulder through the range of motion without resistance.

MMT

## Gravity Minimized

**Patient position:** Sitting with the arm supported on a table in 90 degrees of shoulder abduction and with the elbow in flexion.

**Stabilization:** The clinician stabilizes the scapula on the tested side.

- Grades 2/5 to −2/5: See Figure 6-45

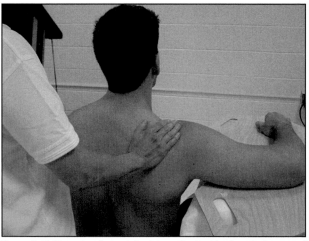

**Figure 6-45**. The patient horizontally abducts the shoulder through the range of motion.

- Grades 1/5 to 0/5: See Figure 6-46

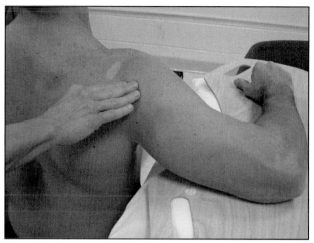

**Figure 6-46**. The posterior deltoid is palpated just below and lateral to the spine of the scapula as the patient attempts to horizontally abduct the shoulder.

**Substitutions:** The patient may extend the elbow when substituting with the triceps brachii or rotate the trunk during testing.

## Horizontal Adduction

### Active Range of Motion

- 0 degrees to 90 degrees (from neutral)

### Prime Movers

- Pectoralis major

  ☐ Origin:

  o Clavicular head: Anterior surface of the medial half of the clavicle

  o Sternal head: Anterior surface of the sternum, the costal cartilages of the upper 6 pairs of ribs, and the aponeurosis of the obliquus externus abdominis

  ☐ Insertion:

  o Clavicular head: Inferior crest of the greater tubercle of the humerus

  o Sternal head: Superior crest of the greater tubercle of the humerus

  ☐ Innervation: Medial pectoral nerve (C6 to T1)

  ☐ Other actions: Internal rotation of the shoulder; clavicular head: flexion of the shoulder; sternal head: extension of the shoulder and anterior tilting of the scapula

  ☐ Palpation site: Anterior axillary fold

### Secondary movers

- Anterior deltoid
- Coracobrachialis
- Biceps brachii

### Anti-Gravity

**Patient position:** Supine with the shoulder in 90 degrees abduction and neutral rotation, elbow flexed to 90 degrees.

**Stabilization:** Weight of the trunk against the table.

MMT

- Grades 5/5 to +3/5: See Figure 6-47

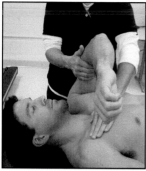

**Figure 6-47**. Resistance is applied to the anterior medial aspect of the arm just proximal to the elbow.

PATIENT DIRECTIVE: *"Move your arm across your chest and do not let me pull it back."*

- Grade 3/5 to +2/5: See Figure 6-48

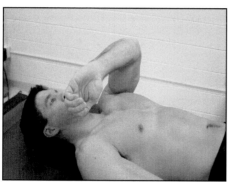

**Figure 6-48**. The patient horizontally adducts the shoulder through the maximal range of motion without resistance.

## Gravity Minimized

**Patient position:** Sitting with the shoulder supported on a table, abducted to 90 degrees, and in neutral rotation with the elbow flexed to 90 degrees.

**Stabilization:** The clinician stabilizes the contralateral shoulder.

MMT

- Grade 2/5 to −2/5: See Figure 6-49

**Figure 6-49**. The patient horizontally adducts the shoulder through the range of motion.

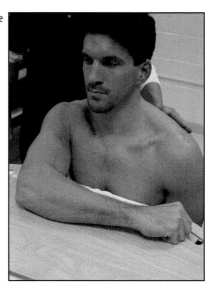

- Grades 1/5 to 0/5: See Figure 6-50

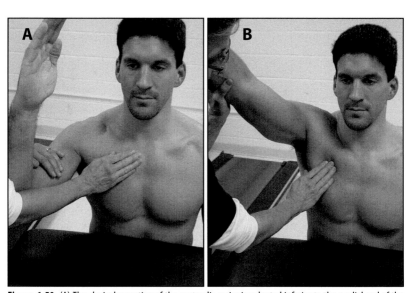

**Figure 6-50.** (A) The clavicular portion of the pectoralis major is palpated inferior to the medial end of the clavicle. (B) The sternal portion is palpated near the anterior axillary fold as the patient attempts to horizontally adduct and extend the shoulder.

**Substitutions:** The patient may attempt to rotate the trunk during testing.

**Points of interest:** The pectoralis major is important during supportive activities, such as crutch walking or ambulating in parallel bars. The patient may be unable to touch the opposite shoulder or reach across the chest, such as when trying to put a seatbelt on, if the pectoralis muscle is weak.

MMT

# Internal (Medial) Rotation

## Active Range of Motion

- 0 degrees to 90 degrees

## Prime Movers

- Subscapularis
  - ☐ Origin: Subscapular fossa
  - ☐ Insertion: Lesser tubercle of the humerus
  - ☐ Innervation: Subscapular nerve (C5 to C6)
  - ☐ Other actions: Slight adduction of the shoulder
  - ☐ Palpation site: On the lateral border of the costal surface of the scapula just deep to the latissimus dorsi muscle

## Secondary Movers

- Pectoralis major
- Teres major
- Latissimus dorsi

## Anti-Gravity

**Patient position:** Prone with the shoulder abducted to 90 degrees and the elbow flexed over the edge of the table. The head should be rotated to the tested side.

**Stabilization:** The clinician stabilizes the humerus and thorax.

MMT

• Grades 5/5 to +3/5: See Figure 6-51

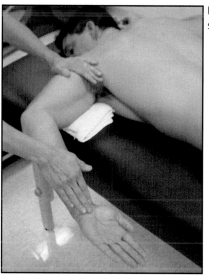

**Figure 6-51**. Resistance is applied to the flexor surface of the forearm just proximal to the wrist.

PATIENT DIRECTIVE: *"Move your arm and hand up toward the ceiling and hold it. Do not let me push it down."*

• Grades 3/5 to +2/5: See Figure 6-52

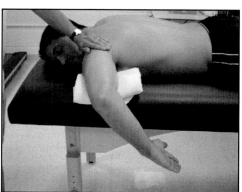

**Figure 6-52**. The patient internally rotates the shoulder through the maximal range of motion without resistance.

## Gravity Minimized

**Patient position:** Prone with the tested arm hanging freely over the edge of the table with the palm facing the table. The head should be rotated to the tested side.

**Stabilization:** The weight of the trunk on the table.

- Grades 2/5 to –2/5: See Figure 6-53

**Figure 6-53.** The patient internally rotates the shoulder so that the palm faces away from the table. The thumb should initiate the movement.

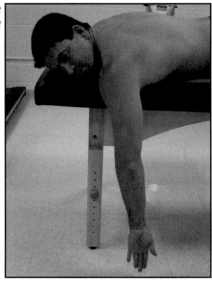

- Grades 1/5 to 0/5: See Figure 6-54

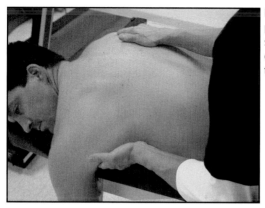

**Figure 6-54.** The subscapularis is palpated on the costal surface of the scapula just deep to the latissimus dorsi muscle as the patient attempts to internally rotate the shoulder.

**Points of interest:** The subscapularis is the only pure internal rotator of the shoulder and is most active when lifting the hand away from the back, such as when tucking a shirt into a pair of pants or when hooking a bra.

MMT

# External (Lateral) Rotation

## Active Range of Motion

- 0 degrees to 90 degrees

### Prime Movers

- Infraspinatus
    - ☐ Origin: Infraspinatus fossa of the scapula
    - ☐ Insertion: Posterior on the greater tubercle of the humerus
    - ☐ Innervation: Suprascapular nerve (C5 to C6)
    - ☐ Other actions: Slight extension of the shoulder
    - ☐ Palpation site: Inferior to the spine of the scapula
- Teres minor
    - ☐ Origin: Upper portion of the lateral border of the scapula
    - ☐ Insertion: Inferior on the posterior aspect of the greater tubercle of the humerus
    - ☐ Innervation: Axillary nerve (C5 to C6)
    - ☐ Other actions: Slight extension of the shoulder
    - ☐ Palpation site: Lateral border of the scapula superior to the inferior angle of the scapula

### Secondary Movers

- Posterior deltoid

### Anti-Gravity

**Patient position:** Prone with the shoulder abducted to 90 degrees and the elbow flexed over the edge of the table. The head should be rotated to the tested side.

**Stabilization:** The clinician stabilizes the humerus and thorax.

MMT

- Grades 5/5 to +3/5: See Figure 6-55

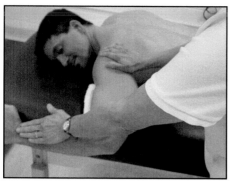

**Figure 6-55**. Resistance is applied to the extensor surface of the forearm just proximal to the wrist.

PATIENT DIRECTIVE: *"Move your arm and the back of your hand up toward the ceiling and hold it. Do not let me push it down."*

- Grades 3/5 to +2/5: See Figure 6-56

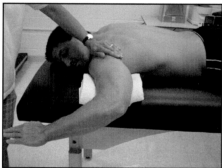

**Figure 6-56**. The patient externally rotates the shoulder through the maximal range of motion without resistance.

## Gravity Minimized

**Patient position:** Prone with the tested arm hanging freely over the edge of the table with the palm facing the table. The head should be rotated to the tested side.

**Stabilization:** The weight of the trunk on the table.

- Grades 2/5 to −2/5: See Figure 6-57

**Figure 6-57.** The patient externally rotates the shoulder so that the palm moves away from the table. The thumb should initiate the movement.

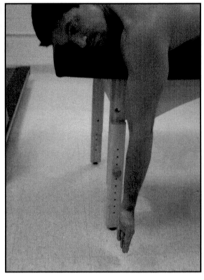

• Grades 1/5 to 0/5: See Figure 6-58

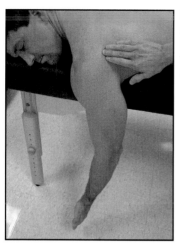

**Figure 6-58.** The infraspinatus is palpated inferiorly to the spine of the scapula and the teres minor is palpated along the lateral border of the scapula superior to the inferior angle of the scapula as the patient attempts to externally rotate the shoulder. (Shown: Palpating the teres minor.)

**Points of interest:** The external rotators of the shoulder are functionally associated with the supinators of the forearm when the elbow is in extension, such as when using a screwdriver or installing a lightbulb into a socket on the ceiling.

MMT

## Scaption

### Active Range of Motion

- 0 degrees to 180 degrees

### Prime Movers

- Supraspinatus
  - ☐ Origin: Supraspinatus fossa of the scapula
  - ☐ Insertion: Superior surface of the greater tubercle of the humerus
  - ☐ Innervation: Suprascapular nerve (C4 to C6)
  - ☐ Other actions: Abduction of the shoulder
  - ☐ Palpation site: Above the spine of the scapula with the shoulder in approximately 30 degrees of shoulder flexion in the sagittal plane from the frontal plane
- Anterior deltoid
  - ☐ Origin: Anterior and superior surface of the lateral third of the clavicle
  - ☐ Insertion: Deltoid tuberosity of the humerus
  - ☐ Innervation: Axillary nerve (C5 to C6)
  - ☐ Other actions: Flexion, internal rotation, and horizontal adduction of the shoulder
  - ☐ Palpation site: Inferior to the lateral third of the clavicle
- Middle deltoid
  - ☐ Origin: Superior lateral surface of the acromion process of the scapula
  - ☐ Insertion: Deltoid tuberosity of the humerus
  - ☐ Innervation: Axillary nerve (C5 to C6)
  - ☐ Other actions: Abduction of the shoulder to 90 degrees
  - ☐ Palpation site: Lateral and inferior to the acromion process

MMT

## Secondary Movers

- None

## Anti-Gravity

**Patient position:** Sitting with the arm elevated approximately 30 degrees of shoulder flexion from the sagittal plane into the frontal plane. The thumb should point up to the ceiling.

**Stabilization:** The clinician stabilizes the opposite shoulder.

- Grades 5/5 to +3/5: See Figure 6-59

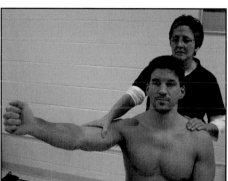

**Figure 6-59.** Resistance is applied just proximal to the elbow joint downward toward the floor.

PATIENT DIRECTIVE: *"Lift your arm halfway between in front of and to the side of you and hold it. Do not let me push it down."*

- Grades 3/5 to +2/5: See Figure 6-60

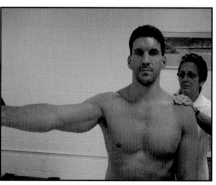

**Figure 6-60.** The patient moves the arm into scaption through the maximal range of motion.

MMT

## Gravity Minimized

**Patient position:** Sitting with the arms by the patient's sides.

**Stabilization:** The clinician stabilizes the opposite shoulder.

- Grades 2/5 to −2/5: See Figure 6-61

**Figure 6-61.** The patient moves the arm through partial range of motion.

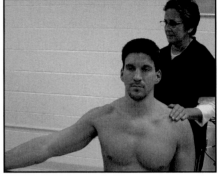

- Grades 1/5 to 0/5: See Figure 6-62

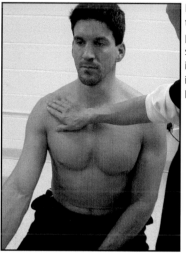

**Figure 6-62.** The anterior deltoid is palpated inferiorly to the lateral third of the clavicle as the patient attempts to perform shoulder scaption. The supraspinatus is palpated superior to the spine of the scapula, with the shoulder in the plane of the scapula, approximately 30 degrees into the sagittal plane from the frontal plane. (Shown: Palpating the anterior deltoid.)

**Points of interest:** The supraspinatus is the muscle most often involved in shoulder "impingement syndrome." It is the major initiator of the first 15 degrees of humeral abduction and serves as a stabilizer for this motion.

MMT

# ELBOW

## Flexion

### Active Range of Motion

- 0 degrees to 145 degrees

### Prime Movers

- Biceps brachii
    - □ Origin:
        - o Short head: Apex of the coracoid process
        - o Long head: Supraglenoid tuberosity at the superior margin of the glenoid
    - □ Insertion: Radial tuberosity and bicipital aponeurosis
    - □ Innervation: Musculocutaneous nerve (C6)
    - □ Other actions: Forearm supination and shoulder flexion
    - □ Palpation site: With the forearm supinated, the belly of the muscle is palpated anteriorly or in the cubital fossa for the tendinous insertion
- Brachialis
    - □ Origin: Distal half of the anterior aspect of the humeral shaft
    - □ Insertion: Ulnar tuberosity and the anterior surface of the corocoid process
    - □ Innervation: Musculocutaneous and radial nerves (C6)
    - □ Other actions: None
    - □ Palpation site: With the forearm pronated, palpate lateral/medial and deep to the biceps tendon just proximal to the cubital fossa

MMT

- Brachioradialis

    □ Origin: Proximal two-thirds of the lateral supracondylar ridge of the humerus

    □ Insertion: Base of the styloid process of the radius

    □ Innervation: Radial nerve (C6 to C7)

    □ Other actions: None

    □ Palpation site: With the forearm midway between pronation and supination and with the elbow flexed to 90 degrees, palpate just lateral to the biceps tendon at the level of or proximal to the elbow joint

### Secondary Movers

- Pronator teres
- Extensor carpi radialis longus
- Flexor carpi radialis
- Flexor carpi ulnaris

### Anti-Gravity

**Patient position:** Sitting, with the elbow flexed to 90 degrees and the forearm supinated (biceps brachii), pronated (brachialis), or in neutral (brachioradialis), depending on which muscle is being tested. General elbow flexion is tested with the forearm in supination.

**Stabilization:** The clinician stabilizes the upper arm against the trunk.

MMT

• Grades 5/5 to +3/5: See Figure 6-63

**Figure 6-63**. Resistance is applied on the anterior forearm just proximal to the wrist.

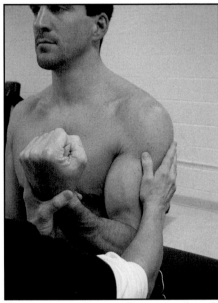

PATIENT DIRECTIVE: *"Bend your elbow up. Do not let me pull your arm down."*

• Grades 3/5 to +2/5: See Figure 6-64

**Figure 6-64**. The patient flexes the elbow through the maximal available range of motion without resistance.

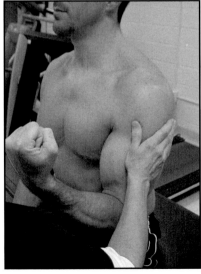

## Gravity Minimized

**Patient position:** Sitting, with the upper extremity resting on a smooth surface. The shoulder should be in 90 degrees of abduction with the elbow in maximal extension and the forearm in neutral rotation.

**Stabilization:** The clinician stabilizes the upper arm against the testing surface.

- Grades 2/5 to –2/5: See Figure 6-65

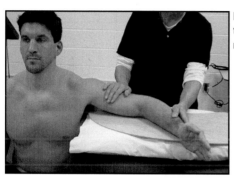

**Figure 6-65**. The patient flexes the elbow through the maximal available range of motion.

- Grades 1/5 to 0/5: See Figure 6-66

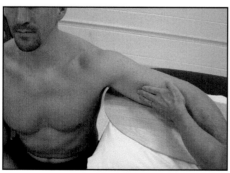

**Figure 6-66**. The elbow flexors are palpated on the anterior aspect of the arm just proximal to the joint as the patient attempts to flex the elbow.

**Substitutions:** The patient may extend the shoulder to cause passive flexion to occur or pronate the forearm or flex the wrist during the attempt to flex the elbow.

**Points of interest:** Rupture of the biceps brachii is often associated with increased age and lifting and is referred to as a "popeye" muscle. Performing a chin-up with the forearm in pronation is more difficult because it places the biceps brachii at a mechanical disadvantage. Of the 3 primary movers, the brachialis is the strongest elbow flexor.

MMT

# Extension

## Active Range of Motion

- 145 degrees to 0 degrees (from maximal elbow flexion)

## Prime Movers

- Triceps brachii

  □ Origin:

    o Long head: Infraglenoid tubercle of the scapula

    o Lateral head: Lateral and proximal surface of the upper one-half of the humeral shaft above the radial groove

    o Medial head: Distal two-thirds of the medial and proximal aspects of the humerus below the radial groove

  □ Insertion

    o All 3 heads insert onto the olecranon process of the ulna

  □ Innervation: Radial nerve (C7 to C8)

  □ Other actions: Extension of the shoulder

  □ Palpation site

    o Long head: Proximal aspect is palpated as it emerges under the posterior deltoid

    o Lateral head: Distal to the posterior deltoid

    o Medial head: Distal on the posterior arm on either side of the common triceps tendon

- Anconeus

  □ Origin: Lateral humeral epicondyle

  □ Insertion: Lateral surface of the olecranon process and upper posterior shaft of the ulna

  □ Innervation: Radial nerve (C7 to C8)

  □ Other actions: Abduction of the ulna during pronation

  □ Palpation site: Deep to the tendinous sheath of the triceps between the lateral epicondyle and olecranon process of the ulna

MMT

## Secondary Movers

- None

## Anti-Gravity

**Patient position:** Supine on a table with the shoulder flexed to 90 degrees and the elbow in maximal flexion.

**Stabilization:** The clinician stabilizes the upper arm.

- Grades 5/5 to +3/5: See Figure 6-67

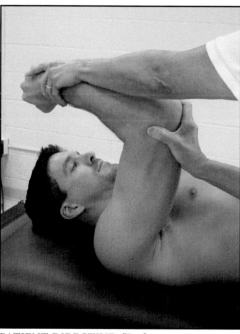

**Figure 6-67.** The patient extends the elbow as resistance is applied just proximal to the wrist on the proximal forearm.

PATIENT DIRECTIVE: *"Push your arm up toward the ceiling and hold it. Do not let me push it down."*

- Grades 3/5 to +2/5: See Figure 6-68

**Figure 6-68.** The patient extends the elbow through the maximal available range of motion without resistance.

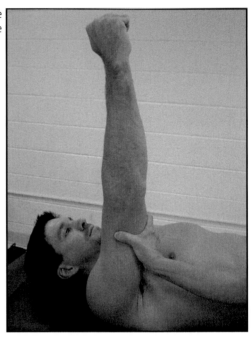

## Gravity Minimized

**Patient position:** Sitting with the upper extremity resting on a smooth surface. The shoulder should be in 90 degrees of abduction and internally rotated with the elbow in maximal flexion and forearm in neutral or pronated.

**Stabilization:** The clinician stabilizes the upper arm.

MMT

- Grades 2/5 to −2/5: See Figure 6-69

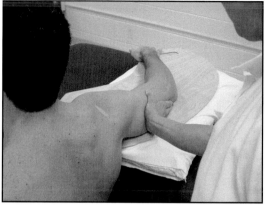

**Figure 6-69**. The patient extends the elbow through maximal range of motion without resistance.

- Grades 1/5 to 0/5: See Figure 6-70

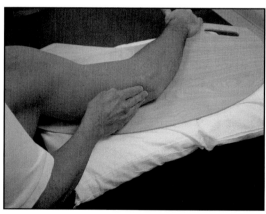

**Figure 6-70**. The elbow extensors are palpated on the posterior aspect of the arm just proximal to the olecranon.

**Substitutions:** The patient may attempt to externally rotate or horizontally adduct the shoulder to substitute for a weak triceps brachii muscle.

MMT

# FOREARM

## Supination

### Active Range of Motion

- 0 degrees to 90 degrees

### Prime Movers

- Supinator

  □ Origin: Lateral epicondyle of the humerus, spinator crest of the ulna, and radial collateral and annular ligaments

  □ Insertion: Lateral surface of the upper third of the radial shaft

  □ Innervation: Radial nerve (C6 to C7)

  □ Other actions: None

  □ Palpation site: Distal to the head of the radius on the dorsal aspect of the forearm, under the common extensor muscles off the lateral epicondyle

### Secondary Movers

- Biceps brachii

### Anti-Gravity

**Patient position:** Sitting with the arm at the patient's side, elbow flexed to 90 degrees, and the forearm in pronation. The fingers should be relaxed.

**Stabilization:** The clinician stabilizes the upper arm against the trunk.

- Grades 5/5 to +3/5: See Figure 6-71

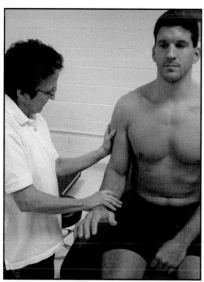

**Figure 6-71**. Resistance is applied to the wrist just proximal to the joint line into pronation.

PATIENT DIRECTIVE: *"Turn your palm up and hold it. Do not let me push it down."*

- Grades 3/5 to +2/5: See Figure 6-72

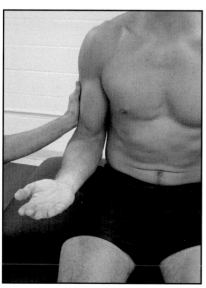

**Figure 6-72**. The patient supinates the forearm through the available range of motion without resistance.

MMT

## Gravity Minimized

**Patient position:** Sitting with the shoulder in approximately 45 degrees of flexion, the elbow flexed, and the forearm in neutral. The clinician supports the arm at the elbow.

**Stabilization:** The clinician stabilizes the upper arm against the trunk.

- Grades 2/5 to –2/5: See Figure 6-73

**Figure 6-73**. The patient supinates the forearm throughout the maximal range of motion.

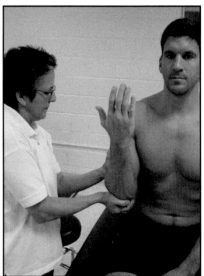

- Grades 1/5 to 0/5: See Figure 6-74.

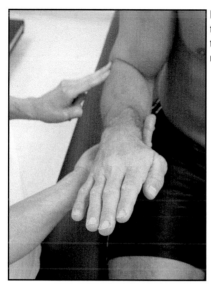

**Figure 6-74**. The supinator is palpated just distal to the head of the radius on the dorsal aspect of the forearm as the patient attempts to perform the movement.

**Substitutions:** The patient may try to externally rotate and adduct the shoulder to passively supinate the forearm. The patient may also extend the wrist.

**Points of interest:** The supinator alone may be active during slow, nonresisted motion. The biceps brachii may be activated to assist if supination with speed or increased resistance is necessary.

## Pronation

### Active Range of Motion

- 0 degrees to 90 degrees

### Prime Movers

- Pronator teres
  - ☐ Origin:
    - o Humeral head: Proximal to the medial epicondyle of the humerus
    - o Ulnar head: Medial aspect of the coronoid process of the ulna
  - ☐ Insertion: Mid-shaft and lateral surface of the radius
  - ☐ Innervation: Median nerve (C6 to C7)
  - ☐ Other actions: Elbow flexion
  - ☐ Palpation site: Medial surface of the cubital fossa to the lateral border of the radius
- Pronator quadratus
  - ☐ Origin: Anterior surface and distal quarter of the ulna
  - ☐ Insertion: Anterior surface and distal quarter of the radius
  - ☐ Innervation: Median nerve (C8)
  - ☐ Other actions: None
  - ☐ Palpation site: Not palpable

### Secondary Movers

- Flexor carpi radialis

### Anti-Gravity

**Patient position:** Sitting with the arm at the patient's side, elbow flexed to 90 degrees, and the forearm in supination. The fingers should remain relaxed.

**Stabilization:** The clinician stabilizes the upper arm against the trunk.

MMT

- Grades 5/5 to +3/5: See Figure 6-75

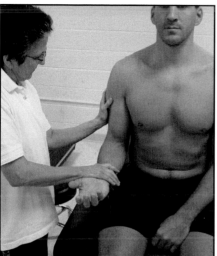

**Figure 6-75.** Resistance is applied to the wrist just proximal to the joint line into supination.

PATIENT DIRECTIVE: *"Turn your palm down and hold it. Do not let me push it up."*

- Grades 3/5 to +2/5: See Figure 6-76

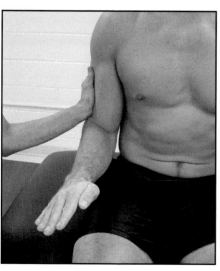

**Figure 6-76.** The patient pronates the forearm through the maximal range of motion without resistance.

MMT

## Gravity Minimized

**Patient position:** Sitting with the shoulder in approximately 45 degrees of flexion, the elbow flexed, and forearm in neutral. The clinician supports the arm at the elbow.

**Stabilization:** The clinician stabilizes the upper arm against the trunk.

- Grades 2/5 to −2/5: See Figure 6-77

**Figure 6-77.** The patient pronates the forearm through the maximal available range of motion.

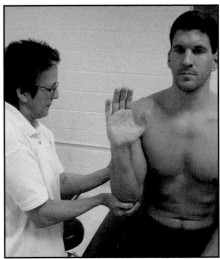

- Grades 1/5 to 0/5: See Figure 6-78

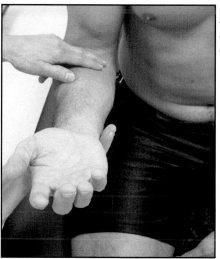

**Figure 6-78.** The pronator teres is palpated on the medial surface of the cubital fossa lateral to the radius as the patient attempts to pronate the forearm.

**Points of interest:** Although both the pronator teres and quadratus are active during pronation of the forearm, the pronator teres becomes more active during explosive activities, such as swinging a raquet or pitching a ball. The pronators are functionally associated with shoulder internal rotation because the 2 motions often occur together during activity.

MMT

# WRIST

## Flexion

### Active Range of Motion

- 0 degrees to 90 degrees

### Prime Movers

- Flexor carpi radialis
  - ☐ Origin: Medial epicondyle of the humerus
  - ☐ Insertion: Base of the second metacarpal bone
  - ☐ Innervation: Median nerve (C6 to C7)
  - ☐ Other actions: Radially deviates the wrist/hand
  - ☐ Palpation site: Slightly lateral to the midline of the wrist
- Flexor carpi ulnaris
  - ☐ Origin
    - o Humeral head: Medial epicondyle from the common flexor tendon
    - o Ulnar head: Medial aspect of the olecranon and proximal border of the ulna
  - ☐ Insertion: Pisiform bone, hamate bone, and base of the fifth metacarpal
  - ☐ Innervation: Ulnar nerve (C7 to C8)
  - ☐ Other actions: Ulnarly deviates the wrist/hand
  - ☐ Palpation site: Immediately proximal to the pisiform

### Secondary Movers

- Palmaris longus
- Flexor digitorum superficialis
- Flexor digitorum profundus
- Abductor pollicis longus
- Flexor pollicis longus

MMT

## Anti-Gravity

**Patient position:** Sitting or supine with the forearm supinated and the dorsal surface resting on a table top. The wrist should be in neutral with the fingers relaxed.

**Stabilization:** The clinician stabilizes the forearm against the table top.

*The flexor carpi radialis and flexor carpi ulnaris may be tested separately by resisting wrist flexion with radial deviation and ulnar deviation, respectively.*

- Grades 5/5 to +3/5: See Figure 6-79

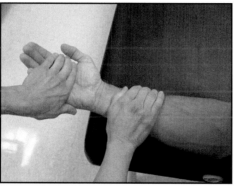

**Figure 6-79.** Resistance is applied to the palm of the hand into wrist extension.

- Grades 3/5 to +2/5: See Figure 6-80

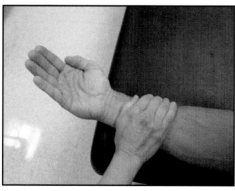

**Figure 6-80.** The patient flexes the wrist straight up without deviation through the maximal available range of motion without resistance.

MMT

## Gravity Minimized

**Patient position:** Sitting or supine with the forearm in neutral and the ulnar border of the hand resting on a table top with the wrist in neutral. The fingers should be relaxed.

**Stabilization:** The clinician stabilizes the forearm against the table top.

- Grades 2/5 to −2/5: See Figure 6-81

**Figure 6-81.** The patient flexes the wrist through the maximal range of motion.

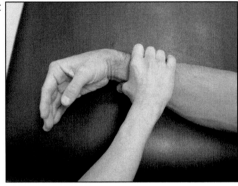

- Grades 1/5 to 0/5: See Figure 6-82

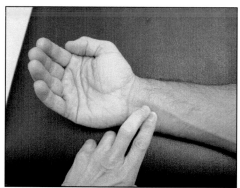

**Figure 6-82.** The flexor carpi radialis is palpated slightly lateral to the midline of the wrist as the patient attempts to flex and radially deviate the wrist. The flexor carpi ulnaris is palpated immediately proximal to the pisiform as the patient attempts to flex and ulnarly deviate the wrist. (Shown: Palpating the flexor carpi radialis.)

**Substitutions:** The fingers may flex as the patient attempts to flex the wrist.

## Extension

### Active Range of Motion

- 0 degrees to 70 degrees

### Prime Movers

- Extensor carpi radialis longus

  □ Origin: Distal third of the lateral supracondylar ridge of the humerus

  □ Insertion: Base of the second metacarpal, dorsal surface

  □ Innervation: Radial nerve (C6 to C7)

  □ Other actions: Radially deviates the wrist/hand

  □ Palpation site: Radiodorsal aspect of the wrist proximal to the second metacarpal

- Extensor carpi radialis brevis

  □ Origin: Lateral epicondyle via the common extensor tendon and radial collateral ligament

  □ Insertion: Base of the third metacarpal bone

  □ Innervation: Radial nerve (C7 to C8)

  □ Other actions: Radially deviates the wrist/hand

  □ Palpation site: In the depression over the capitate bone as the patient abducts the thumb in the sagittal plane

- Extensor carpi ulnaris

  □ Origin: Lateral epicondyle via the common extensor tendon and the posterior aspect of the ulna

  □ Insertion: Medial aspect of the base of the fifth metacarpal bone

  □ Innervation: Radial nerve (C7 to C8)

  □ Other actions: Ulnarly deviates the wrist/hand

  □ Palpations site: The tendon of the extensor carpi ulnaris is palpated on the ulnar side of the dorsal surface of the wrist just distal to the styloid process of the ulna and proximal to the fifth metacarpal

MMT

## Secondary Movers

- Extensor digitorum

- Extensor digiti minimi

- Extensor indicis

## Anti-Gravity

**Patient position:** Sitting with the forearm pronated and supported on a table top. The wrist should be in neutral and the fingers should be relaxed.

**Stabilization:** The clinician stabilizes the forearm against the table top.

*The extensor carpi radialis longus, extensor carpi radialis brevis, and extensor carpi ulnaris may be tested separately by resisting wrist extension with radial deviation and ulnar deviation, respectively.*

- Grades 5/5 to +3/5: See Figure 6-83

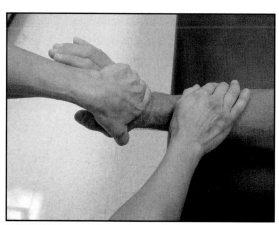

**Figure 6-83.** Resistance is applied to the dorsum of the hand into wrist flexion.

PATIENT DIRECTIVE: *"Move the back of your hand up toward the ceiling and hold it. Do not let me push it down."*

- Grades 3/5 to +2/5: See Figure 6-84

**Figure 6-84.** The patient extends the wrist straight up without deviation through the maximal available range of motion without resistance.

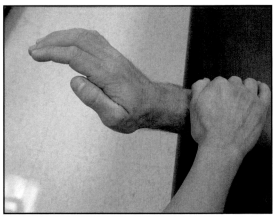

## Gravity Minimized

**Patient position:** Sitting or supine with the forearm in neutral and the ulnar border of the hand resting on a table top with the wrist in neutral. The fingers should be relaxed.

**Stabilization:** The clinician stabilizes the forearm against the table top.

- Grades 2/5 to –2/5: See Figure 6-85

**Figure 6-85.** The patient extends the wrist through the maximal available range of motion.

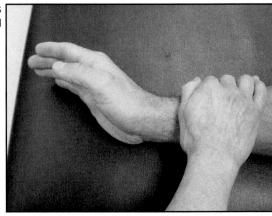

• Grades 1/5 to 0/5: See Figure 6-86

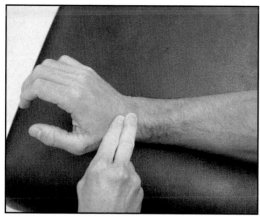

**Figure 6-86.** The extensor carpi radialis longus is palpated on the dorsum of the wrist in line with the second metacarpal, the extensor carpi radialis is palpated on the dorsum of the wrist in line with the third metacarpal, and the extensor carpi ulnaris is palpated on the dorsum of the wrist proximal to the fifth metacarpal just distal to the ulnar styloid process as the patient attempts to extend and radially or ulnarly deviate the wrist, respectively. (Shown: Palpating the extensor carpi radialis longus.)

**Substitutions:** The fingers may extend as the patient attempts to extend the wrist.

MMT

# FINGERS II TO V

*Note:* Because gravity is not a significant factor during testing of the fingers/thumb, the format used for grading muscle strength deviates from the standard grading system applied to other muscle groups; half grades are not assigned.

## MCP Flexion

### Active Range of Motion

- 0 degrees to 90 degrees

### Prime Movers

- Lumbricales

    □ Origin: Originate off of the tendons of the flexor digitorum profundus. Lumbricales #1 and #2: radial sides and plamar surfaces of tendons of digits II and III; #3 is adjacent to sides of digits III and IV; #4 is adjacent to sides of the tendons of digits IV and V

    □ Insertion: Tendinous expansion of the extensor digitorum, with each muscle running distally to the radial side of the corresponding digit and attaching to the dorsal digital expansion

    □ Innervation: Lumbricales #1 and #2; median nerve (C8 to T1) and #3 and #4; ulnar nerve (C8 to T1)

    □ Other actions: Extension of the fingers at the proximal interphalangeal (PIP) and distal interphalangeal (DIP) joints

    □ Palpation site: Not palpable

### Secondary Movers

- Dorsal/palmar interossei

- Flexor digitorum superficialis

- Flexor digitorum profundus

- Flexor digiti minimi

- Opponens digiti minimi

MMT

## GRADES 5/5 (NORMAL), 4/5 (GOOD), AND 3/5 (FAIR)

**Patient position:** Sitting or supine with the forearm in supination and the wrist in neutral. The metacarpophalangeal (MCP) joints should be extended with the PIP and DIP joints flexed.

**Stabilization:** The clinician stabilizes the metacarpal bones against the table top.

- Grades 5/5 to 4/5: See Figure 6-87

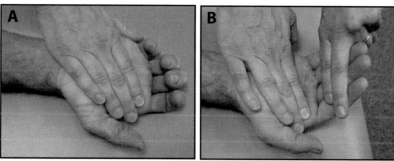

**Figure 6-87.** Resistance is applied to the palmar surface of the proximal row of the phalanges into metacarpophalangeal extension.

PATIENT DIRECTIVE: *"Straighten out your fingers as you bend your hand at the knuckles and hold it. Do not let me push your fingers down."*

*\*The clinician may have to demonstrate the motion first.*

- Grade 3/5: See Figure 6-88

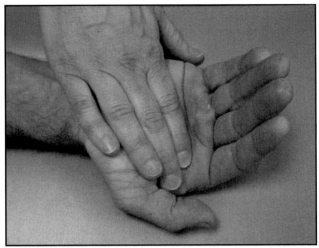

**Figure 6-88.** The patient flexes the metacarpophalangeal joints while simultaneously extending the proximal and distal interphalangeal joints.

## GRADES 2/5 (POOR), 1/5 (TRACE), AND 0/5 (ZERO)

**Patient position:** Sitting or supine with the forearm and wrist in neutral with the hand resting on the ulnar border. The MCP joints should be maximally extended with the PIP and DIP joints in flexion.

**Stabilization:** The clinician stabilizes the wrist and hand.

- Grade 2/5: See Figure 6-89

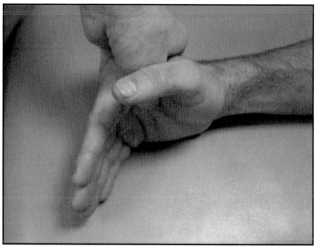

**Figure 6-89.** The patient attempts to flex the metacarpophalangeal joints while simultaneously extending the proximal interphalangeal and distal interphalangeal joints.

*\*The lumbricales are too deep to palpate. A grade of 1/5 or trace is given if any movement is observed and 0/5 is assigned in the absence of movement.*

**Substitutions:** The long finger flexors may cause the PIP and DIP joints to flex as the patient attempts to flex the MCP joints.

MMT

# PIP Flexion

## Active Range of Motion

- 0 degrees to 120 degrees

## Prime Movers

- Flexor digitorum superficialis

  - ☐ Origin: Humero-ulnar head: Medial epicondyle of the humerus and medial aspect of the coronoid process

  - ☐ Radial head: Oblique line of the radius

  - ☐ Insertion: Four tendons insert into each side of the middle phalanx of digits II to V

  - ☐ Innervation: Median nerve (C8 to T1)

  - ☐ Other actions: Assists with flexion of the wrist

  - ☐ Palpation site: The tendons are palpated where they cross the palmar surface of each proximal phalanx

## Secondary Movers

- None

### GRADES 5/5 (NORMAL), 4/5 (GOOD), AND 3/5 (FAIR)

**Patient position:** Sitting or supine with the hand resting on the dorsal side with the wrist in neutral. The tested digit should be slightly flexed at the MCP joint.

**Stabilization:** All joints of the nontested fingers are held in extension.

- Grades 5/5 to 4/5: See Figure 6-90

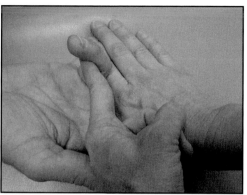

**Figure 6-90**. Resistance is applied to the palmar surface of the middle phalanx of the tested digit into extension.

PATIENT DIRECTIVE: *"Bend your finger and hold it. Do not let me straighten it out. Keep all your fingers relaxed."*

- Grade 3/5: See Figure 6-91

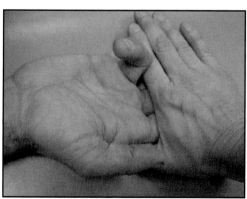

**Figure 6-91**. The patient flexes the proximal interphalangeal of the tested digit through the maximal available range of motion without resistance.

## GRADES 2/5 (POOR), 1/5 (TRACE), AND 0/5 (ZERO)

**Patient position:** Sitting or supine with the forearm in neutral and the ulnar border of the hand resting on a table top.

**Stabilization:** The clinician stabilizes the forearm and holds the nontested digits in extension.

- Grade 2/5: See Figure 6-92

**Figure 6-92.** The patient flexes the proximal interphalangeal joint of the tested digit through the available range of motion.

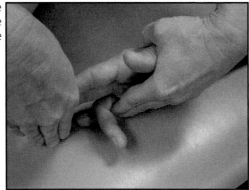

- Grades 1/5 to 0/5: See Figure 6-93

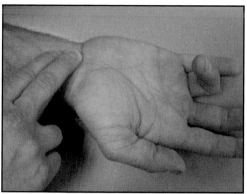

**Figure 6-93.** The flexor digitorum superficialis is palpated on the palmar aspect of the wrist between the palmaris longus and flexor carpi ulnaris.

**Substitutions:** The flexor digitorum profundus may cause flexion of the DIP joints as the patient attempts to flex the PIP joint.

MMT

## DIP Flexion

### Active Range of Motion

- 0 degrees to 80 degrees

### Prime Movers

- Flexor digitorum profundus

  □ Origin: Anterior and medial surfaces of the proximal three-quarters of the ulna

  □ Insertion: Four tendons insert into the base of each distal phalanx of digits II to V

  □ Ulnar nerve, digits IV and V (C8 to T1)

  □ Innervation: Median nerve, digits II and III (C8 to T1)

  □ Other actions: MCP and PIP flexion of fingers II to V. Assists with flexion of the wrist

  □ Palpation site: The tendons are palpated where they cross the palmar surface of each middle phalanx of digits II to V

### Secondary Movers

- None

### Grades 5/5 (normal), 4/5 (good), and 3/5 (fair)

**Patient position:** Sitting or supine with the hand resting on the dorsal surface with the wrist in neutral. The proximal PIP should be in extension.

**Stabilization:** The clinician stabilizes the middle phalanx and PIP joint of the tested digit.

MMT

- Grades 5/5 to 4/5: See Figure 6-94

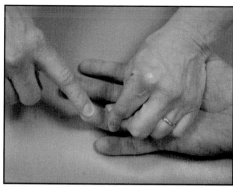

**Figure 6-94**. Resistance is applied to the palmar surface of the distal phalanx into extension.

PATIENT DIRECTIVE: *"Bend the tip of your finger and hold it. Do not let me straighten it out."*

- Grade 3/5: See Figure 6-95

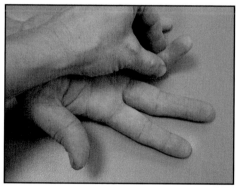

**Figure 6-95**. The patient flexes the distal interphalangeal of the tested digit through the maximal available range of motion without resistance.

MMT

## GRADES 2/5 (POOR), 1/5 (TRACE), AND 0/5 (ZERO)

**Patient position:** Sitting or supine with the forearm in neutral and the ulnar border of the hand resting on a table top.

**Stabilization:** The clinician stabilizes the forearm and holds the middle phalanx of the tested digit in extension.

- Grade 2/5: See Figure 6-96

**Figure 6-96.** The patient flexes the distal interphalangeal joint of the tested digit through the maximal available range of motion.

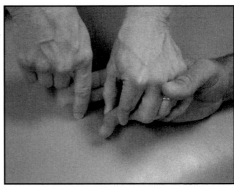

- Grades 1/5 to 0/5: See Figure 6-97

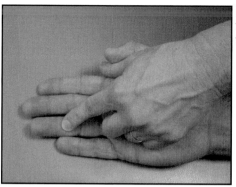

**Figure 6-97.** The flexor digitorum profundus tendons can be palpated on the palmar surfaces of the middle phalanx of digits II to V.

**Substitutions:** The wrist must be kept in a neutral position to prevent tenodesis from occurring from wrist extension.

## MCP Extension

### Active Range of Motion

- 90 degrees to 0 degrees (extension from maximal flexion)
- 0 degrees to 30 degrees (hyperextension)

### Prime Movers

- Extensor digitorum

  □ Origin: Lateral epicondyle of the humerus

  □ Insertion: Via 4 tendons to digits II to V through the extensor hood to the base of the distal phalanx

  □ Innervation: Radial nerve (C7 to C8)

  □ Other actions: Extends the PIP joints of fingers II to V; assists in abduction of fingers I, IV, and V; assists in the extension and abduction of the wrist

  □ Palpation site: Over the dorsal aspect of the hand as the tendons pass down each finger

- Extensor indicis

  □ Origin: Dorsal surface of the shaft of the ulna below the origin of the extensor pollicis longus

  □ Insertion: Second digit extensor hood via the tendon of the extensor digitorum

  □ Innervation: Radial nerve (C7 to C8)

  □ Other actions: Extends the PIP joint of the index finger; assists in adduction of the index finger and in extension of the wrist

  □ Palpation site: Over the dorsal/ulnar aspect of the second metacarpal, close to the hand

MMT

- Extensor digiti minimi

  □ Origin: Lateral epicondyle via the common extensor tendon

  □ Insertion: Extensor hood of the fifth finger with the extensor digitorum

  □ Innervation: Radial nerve (C7 to C8)

  □ Other actions: Extends the PIP joint of the little finger and assists with abduction of the little finger; assists with extension of the wrist

  □ Palpation site: Over the dorsal aspect of the fifth metacarpal, close to the head of the ulna

## Secondary Movers

- None

### Grades 5/5 (normal), 4/5 (good), and 3/5 (fair)

**Patient position:** Sitting or supine with the forearm in pronation and the wrist in neutral with the palmar aspect of the hand resting on a table top and the MCP joints flexed to 90 degrees off the edge of the table.

**Stabilization:** The clinician stabilizes the hand and wrist.

- Grades 5/5 to 4/5: See Figure 6-98

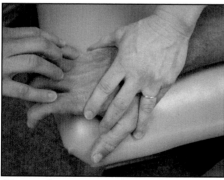

**Figure 6-98.** Resistance is applied to the distal end of the proximal phalanx (dorsally) as the patient extends the MCP joints with the PIP joints in flexion.

*To test the extensor indicis and extensor digiti minimi, the patient extends the MCP joint of the second digit and fifth digit, respectively.*

PATIENT DIRECTIVE: *"Bend your knuckles up and hold it. Do not let me push them down."*

*The clinician may have to demonstrate the motion first.*

MMT

- Grade 3/5: See Figure 6-99

**Figure 6-99.** The patient extends the tested metacarpophalangeal joints through the maximal range of motion without resistance.

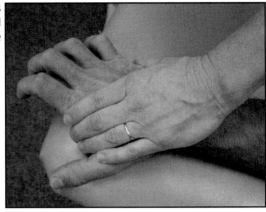

## GRADES 2/5 (POOR), 1/5 (TRACE), AND 0/5 (ZERO)

**Patient position:** Sitting or supine with the forearm and wrist in neutral with the hand resting on the ulnar border on a table top.

**Stabilization:** The clinician stabilizes the hand and wrist.

- Grade 2/5: See Figure 6-100

**Figure 6-100.** The patient extends the metacarpophalangeal joint of the tested digits through the maximal range of motion.

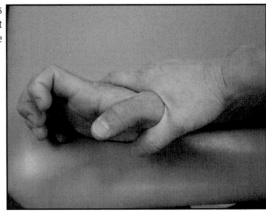

- Grades 1/5 to 0/5: See Figure 6-101

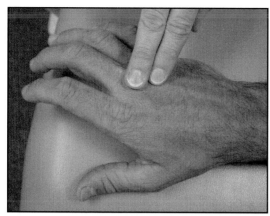

**Figure 6-101**. The tendons of the extensor digitorum, extensor indicis, and extensor digiti minimi are readily palpable on the dorsal surface of the hand as the patient attempts to extend the corresponding metacarpophalangeal joints. (Shown: Palpating the tendons of the extensor digitorum.)

**Substitution:** Flexion of the wrist may cause interphalangeal (IP) extension via tenodesis. Substitution by the lumbricals may also cause extension of the IP joints.

# Finger Abduction

## Active Range of Motion

- 0 degrees to 20 degrees

## Prime Movers

- Dorsal interossei

  - ☐ Origin: Between each metacarpal bone on adjacent sides

  - ☐ Insertion:

    - o First/second: Radial side of the extensor expansion of the second and third digits

    - o Third/fourth: Ulnar side of the extensor expansion of the third and fourth digits

  - ☐ Innervation: Ulnar nerve (C8 to T1)

  - ☐ Other actions: Assists the lumbricals in MCP flexion and PIP/DIP extension of fingers II to V

  - ☐ Palpation site: First dorsal interossei-radial side of the second metacarpal; second dorsal interossei-radial side of the proximal phalanx of the third digit; third dorsal interossei-ulnar side of the proximal phalanx of the third digit; fourth dorsal interossei-ulnar side of the proximal phalanx of the fourth digit

- Abductor digiti minimi

  - ☐ Origin: Pisiform bone and tendon of the flexor carpi ulnaris muscle

  - ☐ Insertion: Base of the proximal phalanx of the fifth digit (ulnar side) and dorsal expansion of the extensor digiti minimi

  - ☐ Innervation: Ulnar side (C8 to T1)

  - ☐ Other actions: Assists with extension of the wrist

  - ☐ Palpation site: Along the ulnar border of the fifth metacarpal

MMT

## Secondary Movers

- Extensor digitorum

- Extensor digiti minimi

### GRADES 5/5 (NORMAL), 4/5 (GOOD), AND 3/5 (FAIR)

**Patient position:** Sitting or supine with the forearm pronated, wrist in neutral, and the palmar aspect of the hand resting on the table top. The fingers should be in extension.

**Stabilization:** The clinician stabilizes the hand and nontested fingers.

- Grades 5/5 to 4/5: See Figure 6-102

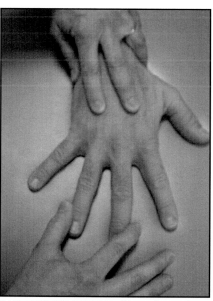

**Figure 6-102.** Resistance is applied to the radial side of one finger and ulnar side of the adjacent finger on the distal end of the proximal phalanx into finger adduction.

PATIENT DIRECTIVE: *"Spread your fingers apart and hold it. Do not let me push them together."*

MMT

- Grade 3/5: See Figure 6-103

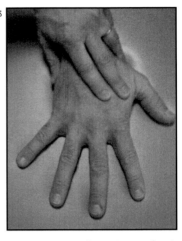

**Figure 6-103**. The patient abducts the tested fingers through the maximal range of motion without resistance.

*\*Because the third digit has 2 dorsal interossei, it is important that it is tested as it moves away from the midline in both directions (ulnarly and radially).*

## GRADES 2/5 (POOR), 1/5 (TRACE), AND 0/5 (ZERO)

**Patient position:** Sitting or supine with the forearm pronated, wrist in neutral, and the palmar aspect of the hand resting on the table. The fingers should be in extension.

**Stabilization:** The clinician stabilizes the hand (and nontested fingers when testing fingers individually).

- Grade 2/5: See Figure 6-104

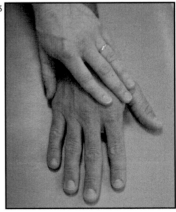

**Figure 6-104**. The patient is able to abduct the tested fingers through partial range of motion.

- Grades 1/5 to 0/5: See Figure 6-105

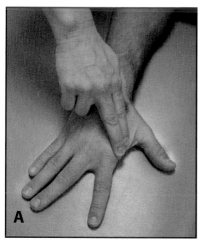 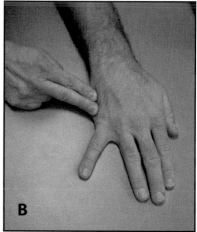

**Figure 6-105.** The dorsal interossei are palpated for the corresponding digit as the patient attempts to abduct the finger. (A) Palpating the first dorsal interossei and (B) palpating the abductor digiti minimi.

*The most readily palpable dorsal interossei muscle is the first, which is located at the base of the proximal phalanx. The abductor digiti minimi is palpated on the ulnar border of the hand as the patient abducts the fifth digit.*

**Substitutions:** The patient may try to extend the MCP joints as they attempt to abduct the fingers.

MMT

# Finger Adduction

## Active Range of Motion

- 0 degrees to 20 degrees

### Prime Movers

- Palmar interossei

  - Origin

    - First: Length of the ulnar side of the second metacarpal

    - Second: Length of the radial side of the fourth metacarpal

    - Third: Length of the radial side of the fifth metacarpal

  - Insertion

    - First: Proximal phalanx, ulnar side of the second digit

    - Second: Proximal phalanx, radial side of the fourth digit

    - Third: Proximal phalanx, radial side of the fifth digit

  - Innervation: Ulnar nerve (C8 to T1)

  - Other actions: Assists the lumbricals in MCP flexion and PIP/DIP extension of fingers II to V

  - Palpation site: First palmar interossei-ulnar side of the proximal phalanx of the second digit; second palmar interossei-radial side of the proximal phalanx of the fourth digit; third palmar interossei-radial side of the proximal phalanx of the fifth digit

### Secondary Movers

- Extensor indicis

## GRADES 5/5 (NORMAL), 4/5 (GOOD), AND 3/5 (FAIR)

**Patient position:** Sitting or supine with the forearm pronated, wrist in neutral, and the palmar aspect of the hand resting on a table top. The fingers should be in extension.

**Stabilization:** The clinician stabilizes the hand and nontested fingers.

MMT

- Grades 5/5 to 4/5: See Figure 6-106

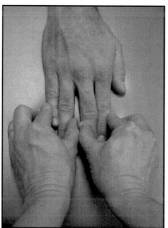

**Figure 6-106**. Resistance is applied to the middle phalanx of each of the 2 adjoining fingers, "pulling" them into abduction.

PATIENT DIRECTIVE: *"Keep your fingers together and do not let me pull them apart."*

*The third digit has no palmar interosseus and is not tested in adduction.*

- Grade 3/5: See Figure 6-107

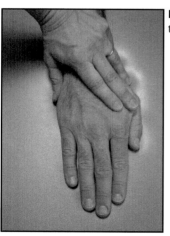

**Figure 6-107**. The patient is able to adduct the fingers toward the middle finger but is unable to hold them against resistance.

MMT

## GRADES 2/5 (POOR), 1/5 (TRACE), AND 0/5 (ZERO)

**Patient position:** Sitting or supine with the forearm pronated, wrist in neutral, and the palmar aspect of the hand resting on a table top. The fingers should be in extension and abducted.

**Stabilization:** The clinician stabilizes the hand and nontested fingers.

•  Grade 2/5: See Figure 6-108

**Figure 6-108.** The patient is able to adduct the tested finger through partial range of motion.

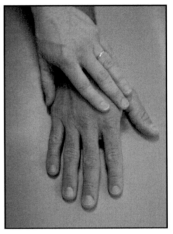

• Grades 1/5 to 0/5: See Figure 6-109

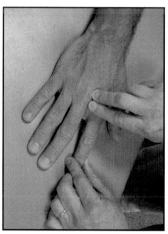

**Figure 6-109**. The palmar interossei are difficult to palpate, but the clinician might be able to detect a slight contraction by placing a finger against the side of the finger to be tested.

**Substitutions:** The patient might flex the fingers while attempting to move them into adduction.

# THUMB

*Note:* Because gravity is not a significant factor during testing of the fingers/thumb, the format used for grading muscle strength deviates from the standard grading system applied to other muscle groups; half grades are not assigned.

## MCP Flexion

### Active Range of Motion

- 0 degrees to 50 degrees (MCP flexion)

### Prime Movers

- Flexor pollicis brevis

    □ Origin: Distal ridge of the trapezium, the trapezoid, capitate, and flexor retinaculum

    □ Insertion: Base of the proximal phalanx of the thumb on the radial side

    □ Innervation: Median nerve (C8 to T1)

    □ Other actions: None

    □ Palpation site: The ulnar side of the first metacarpal

### Secondary Movers

- None

**GRADES 5/5 (NORMAL), 4/5 (GOOD), AND 3/5 (FAIR)**

**Patient position:** Sitting or supine with the forearm in supination, the wrist in neutral, and the hand resting on the dorsal surface on a table top. The thumb is in an adducted position.

**Stabilization:** The clinician stabilizes the first metacarpal.

MMT

- Grades 5/5 to 4/5: See Figure 6-110

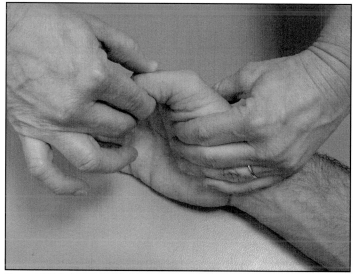

**Figure 6-110.** Resistance is applied to the proximal phalanx into extension.

PATIENT DIRECTIVE: *"Bend the base of your thumb and hold it. Do not let me straighten it out."*

*For a grade of 3/5, the patient flexes the MCP through the maximal range of motion with slight resistance.*

## GRADES 2/5 (POOR), 1/5 (TRACE), AND 0/5 (ZERO)

- Grade 2/5: See Figure 6-111

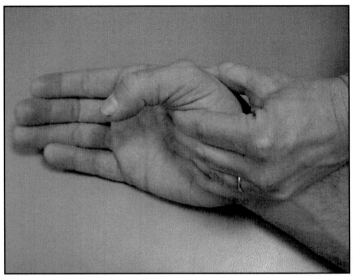

**Figure 6-111**. The patient flexes both the MCP joint of the thumb through maximal range of motion without resistance.

- Grades 1/5 to 0/5: See Figure 6-112

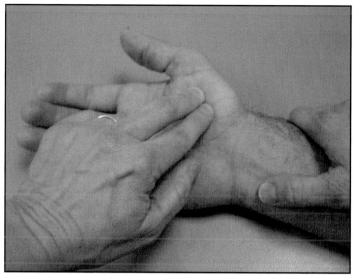

**Figure 6-112**. The flexor pollicis brevis is palpated on the ulnar side of the first metacarpal as the patient attempts to flex the MCP joint.

**Substitutions:** The flexor pollicis longus may be activated to flex the MCP joint. The DIP of the thumb should remain in extension during testing of MCP flexion to avoid this substitution.

# IP Flexion

## Active Range of Motion

- 0 degrees to 90 degrees

### Prime Movers

- Flexor pollicis longus

    ☐ Origin: Anterior surface of the middle half of the shaft of the radius and coronoid process of the ulna

    ☐ Insertion: Base of the distal phalanx of the thumb

    ☐ Innervation: Median nerve (C8 to T1)

    ☐ Other actions: None

    ☐ Palpation site: Palpate where the tendon crosses the palmar surface of the proximal phalanx of the thumb

### Secondary Movers

- None

### GRADES 5/5 (NORMAL), 4/5 (GOOD), AND 3/5 (FAIR)

**Patient position:** Sitting or supine with the forearm in supination, the wrist in neutral, and the hand resting on the dorsal surface on a table top. The thumb is in an adducted position.

**Stabilization:** The clinician stabilizes the proximal phalanx.

- Grades 5/5 to 4/5: See Figure 6-113

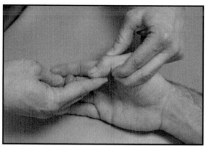

**Figure 6-113**. Resistance is applied to the distal phalanx into extension.

PATIENT DIRECTIVE: *"Bend the tip of your thumb and hold it. Do not let me straighten it out."*

*For a grade of 3/5, the patient flexes the IP joint through the maximal range of motion with slight resistance.*

## GRADES 2/5 (POOR), 1/5 (TRACE), AND 0/5 (ZERO)

- Grade 2/5: See Figure 6-114

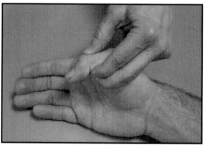

**Figure 6-114**. The patient flexes the IP joint through the maximal range of motion without resistance.

- Grades 1/5 to 0/5: See Figure 6-115

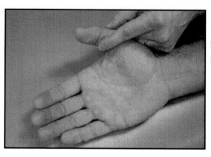

**Figure 6-115**. The tendon of the flexor pollicis longus is palpated where it crosses the palmar surface of the proximal phalanx of the thumb as the patient attempts to flex the IP joint.

MMT

## MCP Extension

### Active Range of Motion

- 50 degrees to 0 degrees (MCP extension)

### Prime Movers

- Extensor pollicis brevis

    □ Origin: Dorsal surface of the distal radius

    □ Insertion: Base of the first proximal phalanx of the thumb

    □ Innervation: Radial nerve (C7 to C8)

    □ Other actions: Assists with wrist radial deviation

    □ Palpation site: Palpate the tendon of the extensor pollicis brevis as it crosses the lateral aspect of the base of the first MCP

### Secondary Movers

- None

**GRADES 5/5 (NORMAL), 4/5 (GOOD), AND 3/5 (FAIR)**

**Patient position:** Sitting or supine with the forearm and wrist in neutral and the hand resting on the ulnar border on a table top.

**Stabilization:** The clinician stabilizes the first metacarpal.

- Grades 5/5 to 4/5: See Figure 6-116

**Figure 6-116.** Resistance is applied to the dorsal surface of the proximal phalanx.

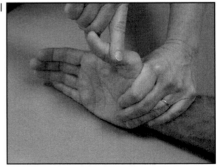

PATIENT DIRECTIVE: *"Straighten your thumb out and hold it. Do not let me push it down."*

*\*For a grade of 3/5, the patient extends the MCP joint through the maximal range of motion with slight resistance.*

MMT

## GRADES 2/5 (POOR), 1/5 (TRACE), AND 0/5 (ZERO)

**Patient position:** Sitting or supine with the forearm and wrist in neutral and the hand resting on the ulnar border on a table top.

**Stabilization:** The clinician stabilizes the first metacarpal.

• Grade 2/5: See Figure 6-117

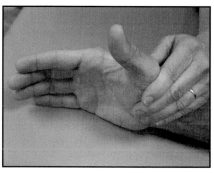

**Figure 6-117**. The patient extends the MCP joint of the thumb through maximal range of motion without resistance.

• Grades 1/5 to 0/5: See Figure 6-118

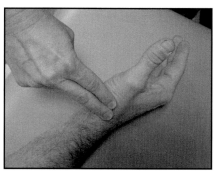

**Figure 6-118**. The extensor pollicis brevis is palpated at the base of the first metacarpal between the tendons of the abductor pollicis and extensor pollicis longus as the patient attempts to extend the first MCP joint. (Shown: Palpating the extensor pollicis brevis.)

**Substitutions:** If the extensor pollicis longus comes into play while the patient is attempting to extend the first MCP joint, the clinician may observe the IP joint of the thumb extend as the carpometacarpal (CMC) joint adducts.

MMT

# IP Extension

## Active Range of Motion

- 90 degrees to 0 degrees

## Prime Movers

- Extensor pollicis longus

    □ Origin: Lateral aspect of the middle third of the dorsal surface of the ulna

    □ Insertion: Base of the first proximal phalanx of the thumb

    □ Innervation: Radial nerve (C7 to C8)

    □ Other actions: Assists with radial deviation

    □ Palpation site: Palpate the tendon of the extensor pollicis longus as it crosses the dorsal aspect at the base of the first MCP

## Secondary Movers

- None

### Grades 5/5 (normal), 4/5 (good), and 3/5 (fair)

**Patient position:** Sitting or supine with the forearm and wrist in neutral and the hand resting on the ulnar border on a table top.

**Stabilization:** The clinician stabilizes the proximal phalanx.

- Grades 5/5 to 4/5: See Figure 6-119

**Figure 6-119.** Resistance is applied to the dorsal surface of the distal phalanx.

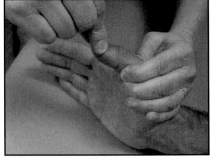

PATIENT DIRECTIVE: *"Straighten the tip of your thumb out and hold it. Do not let me bend it down."*

*For a grade of 3/5, the patient extends the IP joint through the maximal range of motion with slight resistance.*

MMT

## GRADES 2/5 (POOR), 1/5 (TRACE), AND 0/5 (ZERO)

**Patient position:** Sitting or supine with the forearm and wrist in neutral and the hand resting on the ulnar border on a table top.

**Stabilization:** The clinician stabilizes the proximal phalanx and metacarpal.

- Grade 2/5: See Figure 6-120

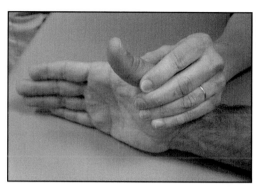

**Figure 6-120.** The patient extends the IP joint through the range of motion without resistance.

- Grades 1/5 to 0/5: See Figure 6-121

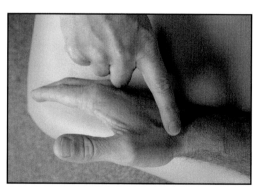

**Figure 6-121.** The extensor pollicis longus is palpated on the ulnar aspect of the "anatomical snuff box" on the dorsal surface at the base of the first metacarpal as the patient attempts to extend the first IP joint.

**Substitutions:** The muscles of the thenar eminence may be activated to flex the CMC joint, resulting in IP joint extension via extensor tenodesis.

MMT

## Thumb Abduction

### Active Range of Motion

- 0 degrees to 60 degrees

### Prime Movers

- Abductor pollicis brevis

  □ Origin: Flexor retinaculum, scaphoid, and trapezium tubercles

  □ Insertion: Base of the first proximal phalanx, radial aspect

  □ Innervation: Median nerve (C8 to T1)

  □ Other actions: None

  □ Palpation site: Along the anterior surface of the shaft of the first meta-carpal

- Abductor pollicis longus

  □ Origin: Lateral aspect of the dorsal surface of the shaft of the ulna

  □ Insertion: Base of the first metacarpal, radial aspect

  □ Innervation: Radial nerve (C7 to C8)

  □ Other actions: Assists with wrist radial deviation

  □ Palpation site: The most anterior of the 3 tendons at the base of the CMC joint; palpate immediately proximal to the CMC joint

### Secondary Movers

- Palmaris longus
- Extensor pollicis brevis
- Opponens pollicis

## GRADES 5/5 (NORMAL), 4/5 (GOOD), AND 3/5 (FAIR)

**Patient position:** Sitting or supine with the forearm supinated and wrist in neutral with the hand resting on the dorsal surface; thumb relaxed into adduction. The MCP and IP joints should be flexed when testing the abductor pollicis longus to decrease thumb extension.

**Stabilization:** The clinician stabilizes the palm of the hand and wrist.

- Grades 5/5 to 4/5: See Figures 6-122

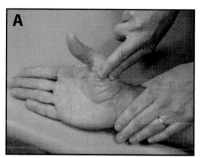 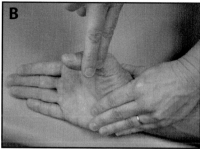

**Figures 6-122.** (A) Resistance is applied to the distal end of the first metacarpal into adduction to test the abductor pollicis longus and (B) the proximal phalanx for the abductor pollicis brevis.

PATIENT DIRECTIVE: *"Move your thumb away from your palm toward the ceiling and hold it. Do not let me push it down."*

- Grade 3/5: See Figure 6-123

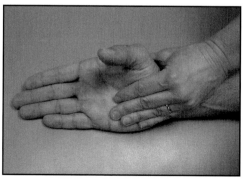

**Figure 6-123.** The patient abducts the thumb through the maximal range of motion without resistance.

MMT

## GRADES 2/5 (POOR), 1/5 (TRACE), AND 0/5 (ZERO)

**Patient position:** Sitting or supine with the forearm in neutral and wrist in neutral with the hand resting on the ulnar border, thumb relaxed into adduction.

**Stabilization:** The clinician stabilizes the palm of the hand and wrist.

- Grade 2/5: See Figure 6-124

**Figure 6-124.** The patient abducts the thumb through maximal range of motion.

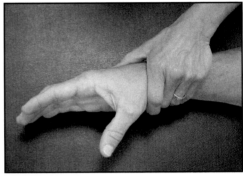

• Grades 1/5 to 0/5: See Figure 6-125

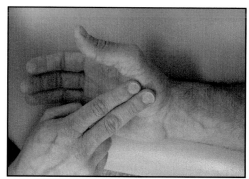

**Figure 6-125.** The abductor pollicis brevis is palpated in the center of the thenar eminence, medial to the opponens, and the abductor pollicis longus is palpated at the base of the first metacarpal on the radial side of the extensor pollicis brevis as the patient attempts to abduct the thumb. (Shown: Palpating the abductor pollicis brevis.)

**Substitution:** If the thumb deviates toward the dorsal surface of the fore-arm, the extensor pollicis brevis is being called in to substitute for the abductor pollicis longus.

*The thumb will deviate radially if the abductor pollicis longus is stronger than the brevis and ulnarly if the abductor pollicis brevis is stronger than the longus.*

MMT

# Thumb Adduction

## Active Range of Motion

- 60 degrees to 0 degrees

## Prime Movers

- Adductor pollicis

    □ Origin: Capitate bone and bases of the second and third metacarpal bones and palmar surface of the distal two-thirds of the third metacarpal bone

    □ Insertion: Ulnar aspect of the base of the proximal phalanx of the thumb

    □ Innervation: Ulnar nerve (C8 to T1)

    □ Other actions: None

    □ Palpation site: Deep in the first web space between the first dorsal interossei and the first metacarpal bone

## Secondary Movers

- First dorsal interosseus

### GRADES 5/5 (NORMAL), 4/5 (GOOD), AND 3/5 (FAIR)

**Patient position:** Sitting or supine with the forearm in pronation and the hand hanging over the edge of a table, supported by the clinician's hand. The wrist is in neutral with the thumb positioned loosely in abduction.

**Stabilization:** The clinician stabilizes the palm of the hand.

- Grades 5/5 to 4/5: See Figure 6-126

**Figure 6-126.** Resistance is applied on the medial aspect of the proximal phalanx of the thumb into abduction.

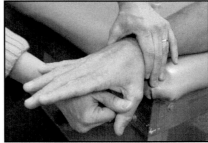

PATIENT DIRECTIVE: *"Move your thumb in toward your index finger and hold it. Do not let me move it out."*

- Grade 3/5: See Figure 6-127

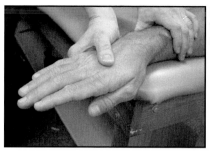

**Figure 6-127.** The patient adducts the thumb through the maximal range of motion without resistance.

## GRADES 2/5 (POOR), 1/5 (GOOD), AND 0/5 (ZERO)

**Patient position:** Sitting or supine with the forearm and wrist in neutral with the ulnar border of the hand resting on the table top with the thumb in abduction.

**Stabilization:** The clinician stabilizes the wrist and hand on the table top.

- Grade 2/5: See Figure 6-128

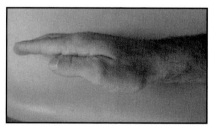

**Figure 6-128.** The patient adducts the thumb through the maximal range of motion.

- Grades 1/5 to 0/5: See Figure 6-129

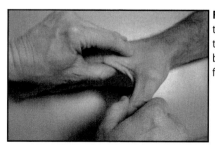

**Figure 6-129.** The adductor pollicis is palpated on the palmar aspect of the first web space between the first dorsal interosseus and the first metacarpal bone by grasping the web space between the index finger and thumb.

MMT

**Substitutions:** The CMC joint will extend if the extensor pollicis longus is activated while the patient attempts to adduct the thumb and flexor pollicis brevis and longus may flex the thumb as the thumb is adducted.

# Thumb Opposition

## Active Range of Motion

- Variable; "normal" range of motion allows for complete motion until the tips of the thumb and fifth digit meet from an open palm position

### Primary Movers

- Opponens pollicis

  □ Origin: Tuberosity of the trapezium and flexor retinaculum

  □ Insertion: Entire lateral aspect of the shaft of the first metacarpal bone

  □ Innervation: Median nerve (C8 to T1)

  □ Other actions: None

  □ Palpation site: Deep to the abductor pollicis brevis along the lateral shaft of the first metacarpal

- Opponens digiti minimi

  □ Origin: Hook of the hamate and flexor retinaculum

  □ Insertion: The entire ulnar margin of the shaft of the fifth metacarpal

  □ Innervation: (C8 to T1)

  □ Other actions: None

  □ Palpation site: Along the shaft of the fifth metacarpal deep to the abductor digiti minimi

### Secondary Movers

- Abductor pollicis brevis
- Flexor pollicis brevis

**GRADES 5/5 (NORMAL), 4/5 (GOOD), AND 3/5 (FAIR)**

**Patient position:** Sitting or supine with the forearm in supination with the wrist in neutral, thumb adducted, and the MCP and IP joints in flexion.

**Stabilization:** The clinician stabilizes the hand and wrist against the table top if necessary.

MMT

- Grades 5/5 to 4/5: See Figure 6-130

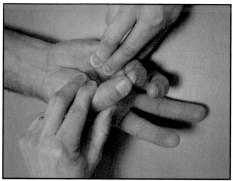

**Figure 6-130.** Resistance is applied at the head of the first metacarpal into lateral rotation, extension, and adduction to test the opponens pollicis and the palmar surface of the fifth metacarpal (trying to "flatten" the palm) for the opponens digiti minimi.

PATIENT DIRECTIVE: *"Put the pads of your thumb and little finger together so they meet in the shape of an 'O' and do not let me pull them apart."*

- Grade 3/5: See Figure 6-131

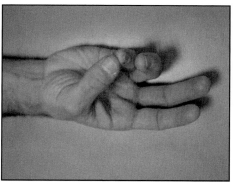

**Figure 6-131.** The patient is able to move the thumb away from the palm and rotate it so that the pad of the thumb touches the pad of the fifth digit.

## GRADES 2/5 (POOR), 1/5 (TRACE), AND 0/5 (ZERO)

**Patient position:** Sitting or supine with the forearm in supination with the wrist in neutral, thumb adducted, and the MCP and IP joints in flexion.

**Stabilization:** The clinician stabilizes the hand and wrist against the table top if necessary.

MMT

- Grade 2/5: Not pictured; the 2 opponens muscles move through the range of motion but are evaluated individually

- Grades 1/5 to 0/5: See Figure 6-132

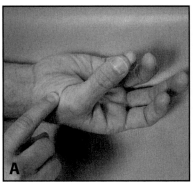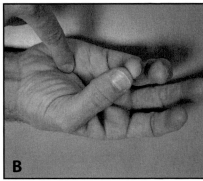

**Figure 6-132.** (A) The opponens pollicis may be palpated along the radial aspect of the first metacarpal, lateral to the abductor pollicis brevis. (B) The opponens digiti minimi may be palpated on the radial aspect of the fifth metacarpal as the patient attempts to oppose the thumb.

**Substitutions:** If the thumb moves parallel to the surface of the palm toward the little finger and touches the tips, not the pads of the fingers, the flexor pollicis longus and brevis have been activated. This is not considered opposition of the thumb.

# SECTION VII

# Trunk/Lower Extremities

Van Ost L, Morogiello J.
*Cram Session in Goniometry and Manual Muscle Testing:*
*A Handbook for Students & Clinicians, Second Edition* (pp 289-375).
© 2023 Taylor & Francis Group.

# TRUNK

## Flexion

### Prime Movers

- Rectus abdominus
  - ☐ Origin: Pubic crest and symphysis
  - ☐ Insertion: Costal cartilage of ribs 5 to 7 and the xiphoid process of the sternum
  - ☐ Innervation: Ventral primary rami (T5 to L1)
  - ☐ Other actions: None
  - ☐ Palpation sites: Upper rectus: both sides of the midline between the umbilicus and xiphoid process; lower rectus: both sides of the midline between the umbilicus and symphysis pubis
- External oblique
  - ☐ Origin: Lateral surface of ribs 5 to 12
  - ☐ Insertion: Linea alba, inguinal ligament, anterior superior iliac spine, pubic tubercle, and anterior half of the iliac crest
  - ☐ Innervation: Ventral primary rami (T5 to L1)
  - ☐ Other actions: Trunk rotation
  - ☐ Palpation site: Opposite side of direction of rotation just below the ribs and lateral to the rectus abdominus
- Internal oblique
  - ☐ Origin: Inguinal ligament, iliac crest, and the thoracolumbar fascia
  - ☐ Insertion: Pubic crest, linea alba, and ribs 10 to 12
  - ☐ Innervation: Ventral primary rami (T7 to L1)
  - ☐ Other actions: Trunk rotation
  - ☐ Palpation site: Just medial to the anterior superior iliac spine along the lateral aspect of the abdomen

## Secondary Movers

- Psoas major

- Psoas minor

## Anti-Gravity

- Upper rectus abdominus

**Patient position:** Supine on a table with both lower extremities in extension.

**Stabilization:** No stabilization of the pelvis is provided if the hip flexors are strong. If weak hip flexors are noted, the clinician stabilizes the pelvis against the table.

- Grade 5/5: See Figure 7-1

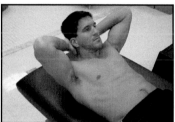

**Figure 7-1.** With the hands clasped behind the head, the patient moves through the range of motion until the inferior angles of the scapulae are off the table. The arms create the resistance.

PATIENT DIRECTIVE: *"Curl your head, shoulders, and torso up until your shoulder blades are off the table."*

- Grades 4/5 and 3/5: See Figures 7-2 and 7-3

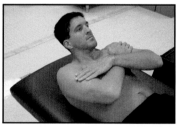

**Figure 7-2.** With the arms crossed over the chest, the patient moves through the range of motion until the inferior angles of the scapulae are off the table for a grade of 4/5.

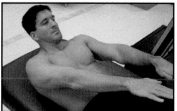

**Figure 7-3.** With the arms fully outstretched over the trunk, the patient completes the range of motion until the inferior angles of the scapulae are off the table for a grade of 3/5.

MMT

**Substitutions:** The patient may rise up rapidly to use momentum to lift the trunk or use their arms to push off the table top. If the patient inhales deeply, it may cause depression of the lower thorax. The umbilicus may deviate to the stronger side.

## Gravity Minimized

- Upper rectus abdominis

**Patient position:** Supine on a table with the knees flexed.

**Stabilization:** The clinician stabilizes the patient's pelvis against the table.

- Grade 2/5: See Figure 7-4

**Figure 7-4.** The patient is able to raise their head against gravity.

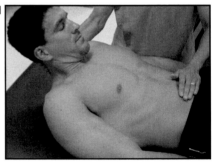

- Grade 1/5: See Figure 7-5

**Figure 7-5.** If there is no depression of the rib cage but there is visable muscle activity noted, contraction of the upper rectus abdominis is palpated on both sides of the midline between the umbilicus and xiphoid process.

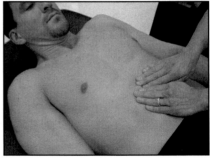

## Anti-Gravity

- Lower rectus abdominus

**Patient position:** Supine on a table with both knees flexed.

**Stabilization:** The weight of the pelvis and lower extremities provide the necessary stabilization. See Figure 7-6.

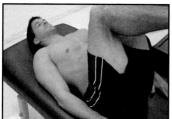

**Figure 7-6.** The patient is able to bring both knees toward the chest and lift the sacrum through the maximal range of motion 10 times for a grade of 5/5 and 4 to 6 times for a grade of 4/5. A grade of 3/5 is assigned if the patient can only complete the motion once.

PATIENT DIRECTIVE: *"Lift both your knees toward your chest and lift your buttocks off the table."*

**Substitutions:** The patient may use the arms to push up or use momentum to lift up the sacrum. The umbilicus may deviate to the stronger side.

## Gravity Minimized

- Lower rectus abdominis

**Patient position:** Supine on a table with the knees flexed.

**Stabilization:** The weight of the trunk and lower extremities stabilizes the patient's pelvis against the table. See Figures 7-7 and 7-8.

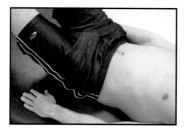 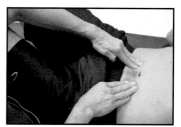

**Figure 7-7.** Patient is able to perform a pelvic tilt for a grade of 2/5.

**Figure 7-8.** Contraction of the lower rectus abdominis is palpated on both sides of the midline between the umbilicus and symphysis pubis for a grade of 1/5.

**Points of interest:** The rectus abdominis and internal and external obliques act together to stabilize the pelvis and contribute to proper postural alignment. Weakness of the abdominal obliques may decrease respiratory efficiency and reduce support of the abdominal viscera.

MMT

## Rotation

### Prime Movers

- External oblique

  □ Origin: Lateral surface of ribs 5 to 12

  □ Insertion: Linea alba, inguinal ligament, anterior superior iliac spine, pubic tubercle, and anterior half of the iliac crest

  □ Innervation: Ventral primary rami of T7 to L1

  □ Other actions: Trunk flexion

  □ Palpation site: Below the ribs and costal cartilages of the lowest ribs in the midclavicular line

- Internal oblique

  □ Origin: Inguinal ligament, iliac crest, and the thoracolumbar fascia

  □ Insertion: Pubic crest, linea alba, and ribs 10 to 12

  □ Innervation: Ventral primary rami of T7 to L1

  □ Other actions: Trunk flexion

  □ Palpation site: Immediately medial to the anterior superior iliac spine along the midclavicular line

### Secondary Movers

- None

### Anti-Gravity

**Patient position:** Supine on a table with the lower extremities extended.

**Stabilization:** The clinician stabilizes the pelvis against the table.

MMT

The scapula corresponding to the external oblique must clear the table for a grade of 5/5. See Figure 7-9.

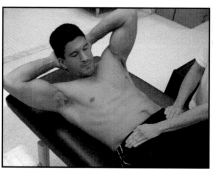

**Figure 7-9.** With the hands clasped behind the head, the patient flexes the trunk and rotates to one side first and then to the opposite side.

PATIENT DIRECTIVE: *"Lift your head and shoulders off the table and turn to your left elbow toward your right knee."*

- Grades 4/5 and 3/5: See Figures 7-10 and 7-11

*Instruct the patient to turn the right elbow toward the left knee to test the opposite side/musculature. When moving the right elbow toward the left knee, the right external and left internal obliques are tested.*

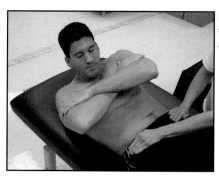

**Figure 7-10.** The patient completes the movement with the hands crossed over the chest for a grade of 4/5.

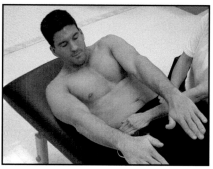

**Figure 7-11.** The patient completes the movement with the arms outstretched in front of the body for a grade of 3/5.

MMT

**Substitutions:** The pectoralis major may cause the shoulders to shrug or slightly lift the shoulder off the table.

## Gravity Minimized

**Patient position:** Supine on the table with the lower extremities extended.

**Stabilization:** The clinician stabilizes the pelvis against the table. See Figure 7-12.

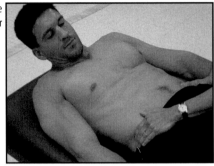

**Figure 7-12.** The patient is able to initiate the elevation of the opposite scapula with the upper extremities by the sides for a grade of +2/5.

- Grades 1/5 to 0/5: See Figure 7-13.

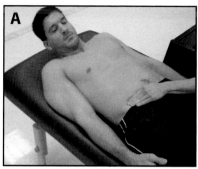 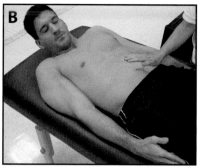

**Figures 7-13.** (A) The internal obliques are palpated on the side toward which the patient turns just medial to the ASIS on the lateral aspect of the abdomen. (B) The external obliques are palpated on the side away from the direction of turning just below the ribs and lateral to the rectus abdominus.

*The umbilicus will move toward the strongest quadrant when there is unequal strength in the opposing obliques.*

*Note:* The direction of the muscle fibers of the internal obliques can be mimicked by crossing the arms over the abdomen and placing the fingertips on each anterior superior iliac spine. The fingers will parallel the muscle fibers (up and in). The direction of the muscle fibers of the external obliques can be mimicked by positioning the hands into the pants pockets (down and in).

MMT

# Extension

## Prime Movers

*Note:* Palpation sites are not listed as the individual muscles cannot be isolated.

- Iliocostalis thoracis
  - Origin: Angles of ribs 7 to 12
  - Insertion: Angles of ribs 6 to 1 and the transverse process of C7
  - Innervation: Dorsal primary rami of the thoracic spinal nerves
  - Other actions: Trunk lateral flexion
- Longissimus thoracis
  - Origin: Lumbar transverse processes (L1 to L5) and thoracolumbar fascia
  - Insertion: Transverse processes of T1 to T12 and ribs 2 to 12 between the angles and tubercles
  - Innervation: Dorsal primary rami of the thoracic spinal nerves
  - Other actions: None
- Semispinalis thoracis
  - Origin: Transverse processes of T6 to T10
  - Insertion: Spinous processes of C6 to T4
  - Innervation: Dorsal primary rami of the thoracic spinal nerves
  - Other actions: Contralateral trunk flexion
- Multifidi
  - Origin: Articular processes of C4 to C7, transverse processes of T1 to T12, mamillary processes of L1 to L5, sacroiliac ligaments, posterior superior iliac spine, and sacrum
  - Insertion: Spinous process of higher vertebrae (2 to 4 and above)
  - Innervation: Dorsal primary rami of the thoracic and lumbar spinal nerves
  - Other actions: Trunk lateral flexion and trunk rotation

MMT

- Rotatores thoracis and lumborum
  - ☐ Origin: Transverse processes of the thoracic and lumbar vertebrae
  - ☐ Insertion: Lamina of the next highest vertebrae
  - ☐ Innervation: Dorsal primary rami of the thoracic and lumbar spinal nerves
  - ☐ Other actions: Trunk rotation
- Interspinalis thoracis and lumborum
  - ☐ Origin/Insertion
    - ○ Thoracis: Three pairs between the spinous processes of T1 to T2, T2 to T3, and T11 to T12
    - ○ Lumbar: Four pairs between the spinous processes of all 5 lumbar vertebrae
  - ☐ Innervation: Dorsal primary rami of the thoracic and lumbar spinal nerves
  - ☐ Other actions: None
- Intertransversarii thoracis and lumborum
  - ☐ Origin/Insertion
    - ○ Thoracis: Eleven pairs between spinous processes of T1 to T12
    - ○ Lumbar: Four pairs between spinous processes of L1 to L5
  - ☐ Innervation: Dorsal primary rami of the thoracic and lumbar spinal nerves
  - ☐ Other actions: Trunk lateral flexion
- Quadratus lumborum
  - ☐ Origin: Iliolumbar ligaments. Iliac crest and superior borders of the transverse processes of L2 to L5
  - ☐ Insertion: Inferior border of the twelfth rib and transverse processes of L1 to L4
  - ☐ Innervation: Ventral primary rami of L1 to L3
  - ☐ Other actions: Pelvic elevation and trunk lateral flexion

MMT

## Secondary Movers

- Gluteus maximus

## Anti-Gravity

- Lumbar

**Patient position:** Prone with the hands clasped behind the head.

*\*Alternate position: Prone with pillows under the patient's hips and the hands clasped on the buttocks.*

**Stabilization:** The clinician stabilizes the pelvis and hips.

PATIENT DIRECTIVE: *"Lift your head and chest up toward the ceiling as high as possible and hold it." See Figures 7-14 and 7-15.*

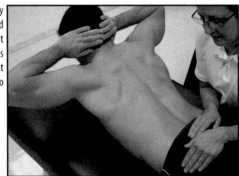

**Figure 7-14.** The patient is able to easily reach the endpoint of the movement and hold it against gravity with minimal effort (grade 5/5). For grade 4/5, the patient is able to reach the endpoint of the movement but demonstrates increased effort trying to maintain the position.

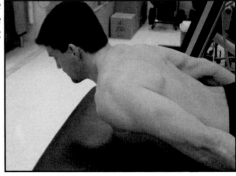

**Figure 7-15.** The patient is able to complete the maximal range of motion (so that the umbilicus clears the table) with the arms at the patient's sides for a grade of 3/5.

## Gravity Minimized

· Lumbar

**Patient position:** Sitting backward on a chair or on a stool with the hands resting on a table top.

**Stabilization:** Achieved by the weight of the patient on the chair and patient compliance. See Figure 7-16.

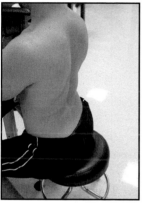

**Figure 7-16.** The patient extends the lumbar spine, anteriorly tilting the pelvis, causing increased lumbar lordosis for a grade of 2/5.

· Grades 1/5 to 0/5: See Figure 7-17

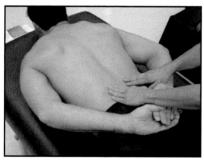

**Figure 7-17.** The lumbar erector spinae musculature is palpated adjacent to both sides of the spine as the patient attempts to extend.

## Anti-Gravity

· Thoracic

**Patient position:** Prone with the head and upper trunk draped at chest level off the edge of a table with the hands clasped behind the head.

*\*Alternate position: Prone with pillows under the abdomen and with the hands clasped on the buttocks.*

MMT

**Stabilization:** The clinician stabilizes the pelvis and lumbar vertebrae.

PATIENT DIRECTIVE: *"Lift your head, shoulders, and chest up toward the ceiling as high as possible and hold it."* See Figures 7-18 and 7-19.

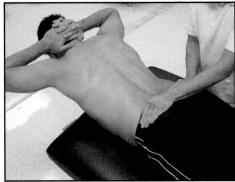

**Figure 7-18.** The patient is easily able to raise the upper trunk so it is at least horizontal to the table top with minimal effort for a grade of 5/5. For grade 4/5, the patient is able to extend the trunk so that it is horizontal to the table level but with some effort.

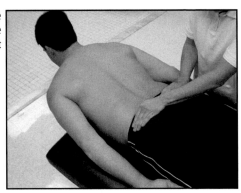

**Figure 7-19.** The patient is able to complete the maximal range of motion so that the umbilicus clears the table with the arms at the patient's sides for a grade of 3/5.

## Gravity Minimized

- Thoracic

**Patient position:** Sitting backward on a chair with the thoracic spine relaxed and the hands resting on the back of the chair.

**Stabilization:** Weight of the patient on the chair and patient compliance. See Figure 7-20.

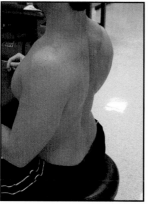

**Figure 7-20.** The patient extends the thoracic and lumbar spine through the maximal range of motion for a grade of 2/5.

• Grades 1/5 to 0/5: See Figure 7-21

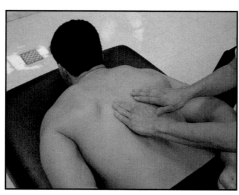

**Figure 7-21.** The thoracic erector spinae musculature is palpated adjacent to both sides of the spine as the patient attempts to extend.

**Substitutions:** The patient may use momentum by forcefully pushing the shoulders backward.

**Points of interest:** The longissimus is the predominant muscle that is active during all motions of the trunk.

MMT

## Pelvic Elevation
### Prime Movers

- Quadratus lumborum

    ☐ Origin: Superior borders of the transverse processes of L2 to L5

    ☐ Insertion: Inferior border of the twelfth rib and transverse processes of L1 to L4

    ☐ Innervation: Ventral primary rami of L1 to L3

    ☐ Other actions: Lateral trunk flexion to the same side. Stabilizes the twelfth rib during inspiration

    ☐ Palpation site: Too deep to be palpated

### Secondary Movers

- Latissimus dorsi
- Iliocostalis lumborum

### Anti-Gravity

**Patient position:** Standing on a stool or step with the clinician supporting the patient for balance, the test limb hanging free.

**Stabilization:** The clinician stabilizes the pelvis on the opposite side.

- Grades 5/5 to 4/5: See Figure 7-22

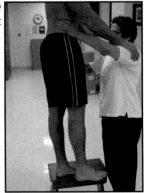

**Figure 7-22.** The patient hikes the hip, elevating the pelvis on the side being tested. Resistance is applied in a downward direction on the iliac crest on the tested side, attempting to laterally tilt the pelvis.

PATIENT DIRECTIVE: *"Hike your hip up toward your ribs and hold it."*

MMT

- Grade 3/5: See Figure 7-23

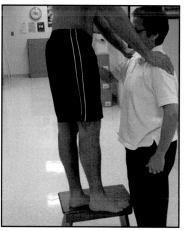

**Figure 7-23.** The patient hikes the pelvis through the range of motion without resistance.

**Substitution:** The patient may laterally flex the trunk away from the tested side.

## Gravity Minimized

**Patient position:** Supine or prone on a table with the lower extremities in extension.

**Stabilization:** The patient may hold onto the sides of the table for resistance.

- Grade 2/5: See Figure 7-24

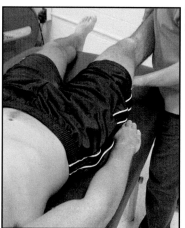

**Figure 7-24.** The patient hip hikes through the available range of motion.

# HIP

## Flexion

### Active Range of Motion

- 0 degrees to 125 degrees (with the knee flexed)

### Prime Movers

- Psoas major
  - ☐ Origin: All lumbar vertebral bodies, transverse processes
  - ☐ Insertion: Lesser trochanter of the femur
  - ☐ Innervation: Spinal nerves of L1 to L3
  - ☐ Other actions: Assists with lumbar flexion and lateral flexion of the trunk
  - ☐ Palpation site: Deep into the abdomen inferior to the ribs and superior to the iliac crest, pushing toward the posterior abdominal wall; the patient must be seated and slightly forward-flexed to relax the abdominal wall
- Iliacus
  - ☐ Origin: Upper two-thirds of the iliac fossa and iliac crest
  - ☐ Insertion: Lesser trochanter of the femur
  - ☐ Innervation: Spinal nerves of L2 to L3
  - ☐ Other actions: None
  - ☐ Palpation site: The iliacus is too deep to palpate accurately

### Secondary Movers

- Rectus femoris
- Sartorius
- Tensor fasciae latae
- Pectineus

- Adductor brevis
- Adductor magnus (superior fibers)
- Gluteus medius (anterior fibers)

## Anti-Gravity

**Patient position:** Seated on the edge of a table with the arms resting by the sides and the hands on the table for stability.

**Stabilization:** The clinician stabilizes the opposite side of the pelvis.

- Grades 5/5 to +3/5: See Figure 7-25

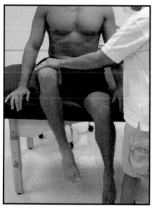

**Figure 7-25**. Resistance is applied over the distal thigh just proximal to the knee joint in a downward direction.

PATIENT DIRECTIVE: *"Raise your knee up toward the ceiling and hold it. Do not let me push it down."*

- Grades 3/5 to +2/5: See Figure 7-26

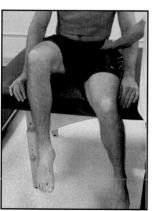

**Figure 7-26.** The patient is able to flex the hip through the maximal range of motion without resistance.

MMT

## Gravity Minimized

**Patient position:** Sidelying with the tested limb resting on a powder board with the hip in neutral and the knee flexed to 90 degrees or with the clinician supporting the tested limb.

**Stabilization:** The clinician stabilizes the opposite side of the hip against the table.

- Grades 2/5 to –2/5: See Figure 7-27

**Figure 7-27.** The patient is able to flex the hip through the maximal range of motion.

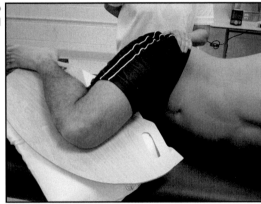

- Grades 1/5 to 0/5: See Figure 7-28

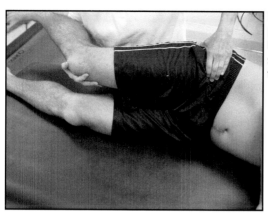

**Figure 7-28.** The hip flexors are palpated just distal to the inguinal ligament on the medial side of the sartorius as the patient attempts to flex the hip.

**Substitutions:** The hip may abduct or externally rotate if the sartorius is activated or abduction with internal rotation may occur if the tensor fasciae latae is activated.

**Points of interest:** Because the psoas major and iliacus share a common insertion and they both flex the hip (and the trunk when the lower extremities are fixed), this muscle group is often referred to as the "iliopsoas." Trauma or retroperitoneal pathology may contribute to weakness of this muscle group.

MMT

# Hip Flexion/Abduction/External Rotation With Knee Flexion

## Prime Movers

- Sartorius
    - ☐ Origin: Anterior superior iliac spine and the upper half of the iliac notch
    - ☐ Insertion: Proximal aspect of the medial tibia
    - ☐ Innervation: Femoral nerve (L2 to L3)
    - ☐ Other actions: Assists with flexion of the knee and internal rotation of the tibia when the knee is flexed in non–weight-bearing
    - ☐ Palpation site: Inferior and slightly medial to the anterior superior iliac spine

## Secondary Movers

- All hip and knee flexors
- All hip abductors and external rotators

## Anti-Gravity

**Patient position:** Sitting on the edge of a table with the arms resting by the sides and the hands on the table for stability.

**Stabilization:** Stabilization is achieved through patient compliance.

- Grades 5/5 to +3/5: See Figure 7-29

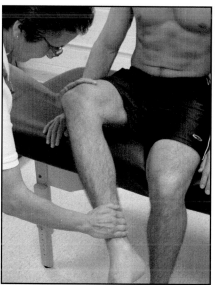

**Figure 7-29.** Resistance is applied to the medial aspect of the ankle (resisting external rotation of the hip) and to the lateral surface of the thigh proximal to the knee (resisting hip flexion and abduction).

PATIENT DIRECTIVE: *"Bring the sole of your foot up toward the opposite knee and hold it. Do not let me move your leg."*

- Grades 3/5 to +2/5: See Figure 7-30

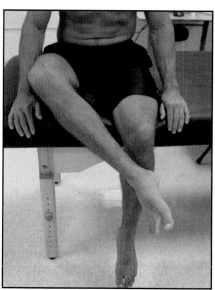

**Figure 7-30.** The patient is able to move the tested hip through the maximal available range of motion without resistance.

MMT

## Gravity Minimized

**Patient position:** Supine with the heel of the tested lower leg on the opposite ankle and the nontested lower leg in extension.

**Stabilization:** Is achieved by the weight of the patient on the table and by patient compliance.

- Grades 2/5 to –2/5: See Figure 7-31

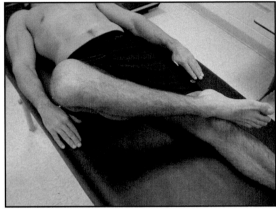

**Figure 7-31.** The patient is able to slide the heel of the tested lower leg up toward the opposite knee.

- Grades 1/5 to 0/5: See Figure 7-32

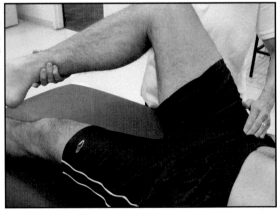

**Figure 7-32.** The sartorius may be palpated just inferior to the anterior superior iliac spine at its origin or on the medial side of the thigh as it crosses over the femur.

MMT

**Substitutions:** If the hip flexes without abduction or external rotation, the iliopsoas and rectus femoris may be substituting for the sartorius. If the hip flexion and abduction occurs with internal rotation, the tensor fasciae latae is being activated.

**Points of interest:** The sartorius derives its name from the Latin word sartor, which means "tailor" because it helps to initiate the action required to cross the legs when sitting. It is the longest muscle in the body and forms the lateral border of the femoral triangle.

# Extension

## Active Range of Motion

- 0 degrees to 15 degrees (hyperextension)

### Prime Movers

- Gluteus maximus

  ☐ Origin: Posterior gluteal line of the ilium, posterior medial aspect of the iliac crest, dorsal aspect of the sacrum, coccyx, and sacrotuberous ligament

  ☐ Insertion: Gluteal tuberosity of the the femur and iliotibial tract

  ☐ Innervation: Inferior gluteal nerve (L5 to S2)

  ☐ Other actions: External rotation of the hip when in extension

  ☐ Palpation site: With the hip positioned in external rotation between the sacrum and greater trochanter

- Semitendinosus

  ☐ Origin: Upper, inferiomedial impression of the ischial tuberosity (with the tendon of the biceps femoris)

  ☐ Insertion: Proximal medial shaft of the tibia and pes anserine

  ☐ Innervation: Tibial division of the sciatic nerve (L5 to S2)

  ☐ Other actions: Knee flexion and internal rotation of the tibia when the knee is flexed

  ☐ Palpation site: Just proximal to the posterior aspect of the knee joint on the medial side

- Semimembranosus

  ☐ Origin: Superolateral aspect of the ischial tuberosity

  ☐ Insertion: Posteromedial aspect of the medial tibial condyle

MMT

- ☐ Innervation: Tibial division of the sciatic nerve (L5 to S2)

- ☐ Other actions: Knee flexion and internal rotation of the tibia when the knee is flexed

- ☐ Palpation site: Just proximal to the posterior aspect of the knee joint on either side of the semitandinosus tendon

- Biceps femoris

  - ☐ Origin

    - o Long head: Ischial tuberosity

    - o Short head: Lateral lip of the linea aspera and the proximal supracondylar line of the femur

  - ☐ Insertion

    - o Fibular head: Lateral tibial condyle

    - o Short head: Peroneal division of the sciatic nerve (L5 to S1)

  - ☐ Innervation: Long head: Tibial division of the sciatic nerve (L5 to S1)

  - ☐ Other actions: Knee flexion, external rotation of the tibia when the knee is flexed

  - ☐ Palpation site: Along the lateral posterior thigh just proximal to the knee joint

## Secondary Movers

- Adductor magnus (inferior fibers)
- Gluteus medius (posterior fibers)

## Anti-Gravity

**Patient position:** Prone on a table with the arms by the sides and the lower extremities extended.

*\*Alternate position: standing with the trunk flexed over a table and with the knee flexed to 90 degrees to isolate the gluteus maximus.*

**Stabilization:** The clinician stabilizes the pelvis against the table.

MMT

• Grades 5/5 to +3/5: See Figure 7-33

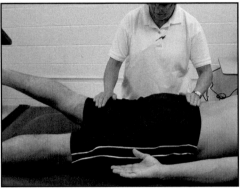

**Figure 7-33.** Resistance is applied on the posterior thigh just proximal to the knee in a downward direction (toward the floor).

PATIENT DIRECTIVE: *"Raise your leg as high as you can toward the ceiling and hold it. Do not let me push it down."*

• Grades 3/5 to +2/5: See Figure 7-34

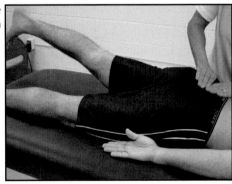

**Figure 7-34.** The patient is able to raise the limb through the maximal range of motion without resistance.

## Gravity Minimized

**Patient position:** Sidelying with the tested limb on top supported on a powder board or by the clinician. The knee is positioned loosely in extension and the bottom hip and knee are flexed for stability.

**Stabilization:** The clinician stabilizes the pelvis against the table.

- Grades 2/5 to –2/5: See Figure 7-35

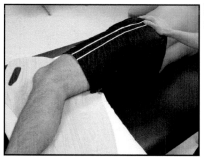

**Figure 7-35.** The patient extends the hip through the maximal range of motion.

- Grades 1/5 to 0/5: See Figure 7-36

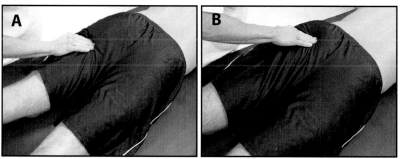

**Figure 7-36.** (A) The proximal hamstrings are palpated at the ischial tuberosity and (B) the gluteus maximus is palpated deep in the center of the buttock.

**Substitutions:** The lumbar spine may extend as the patient attempts to extend the hip joint.

**Points of interest:** The gluteus maximus is the most powerful extensor of the hip. It is primarily active during movements such as stair climbing, rising from a squat to a standing position, and climbing. It is minimally active during normal gait. If there is weakness of the gluteus maximus, a "gluteus maximus lurch" may result. The hamstrings are significant in maintaining hip extension when in standing.

MMT

## Abduction

### Active Range of Motion

- 0 degrees to 45 degrees

### Prime Movers

- Gluteus medius
  - ☐ Origin: Outer surface of the ilium from the iliac crest and posterior gluteal line above to the anterior gluteal line below
  - ☐ Insertion: Lateral surface of the greater trochanter
  - ☐ Innervation: Superior gluteal nerve (L4 to S1)
  - ☐ Other actions: Slight internal rotation of the hip
  - ☐ Palpation site: Just proximal to the greater trochanter and laterally just distal to the iliac crest
- Gluteus minimus
  - ☐ Origin: External surface of the ilium and inferior gluteal line
  - ☐ Insertion: Anterior surface of the greater trochanter
  - ☐ Innervation: Superior gluteal nerve (L4 to S1)
  - ☐ Other actions: Slight internal rotation of the hip
  - ☐ Palpation site: The gluteus minimus lies deep to the gluteus maximus and is not palpable

### Secondary Movers

- Upper fibers of the gluteus maximus
- Tensor fasciae latae
- Obturator internus
- Gemellus superior and inferior
- Sartorius

MMT

## Anti-Gravity

**Patient position:** Sidelying with the bottom hip and knee flexed for stability; the tested limb lies on top with the hip and knee extended and in neutral.

**Stabilization:** The clinician stabilizes the pelvis.

- Grades 5/5 to +3/5: See Figure 7-37

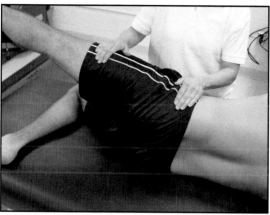

**Figure 7-37.** Resistance is applied on the lateral aspect of the thigh just proximal to the knee joint.

PATIENT DIRECTIVE: *"Raise your leg up toward the ceiling and hold it. Do not let me push it down."*

- Grades 3/5 to +2/5: See Figure 7-38

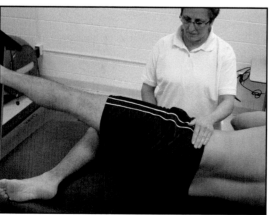

**Figure 7-38.** The patient abducts the hip through the maximal range of motion without resistance.

MMT

## Gravity Minimized

**Patient position:** Supine with the tested limb in extension resting on a smooth surface or supported by the clinician.

**Stabilization:** The clinician stabilizes the pelvis.

- Grades 2/5 to –2/5: See Figure 7-39

**Figure 7-39.** The patient abducts the hip through the available range of motion.

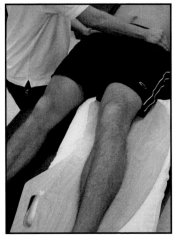

- Grades 1/5 to 0/5: See Figure 7-40

**Figure 7-40.** The gluteus medius is palpated on the lateral aspect of the hip just superior to the greater trochanter as the patient attempts to abduct the hip.

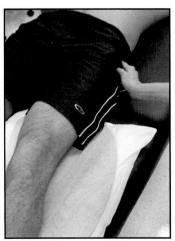

**Substitutions:** The patient's pelvis may elevate (hip hike) if the gluteus medius is weak. The tested hip may externally rotate and flex in an attempt to substitute with the hip flexors.

**Points of interest:** If the gluteus medius and minimus are weak, it will result in a trendelenburg gait pattern. Only these 2 muscles can stabilize the pelvis during single-limb closed-chain movement.

# Abduction From a Flexed Hip

## Prime Movers

- Tensor fasciae latae

  □ Origin: Anterior aspect of the outer lip of the iliac crest and the anterior border of the ilium

  □ Insertion: Lateral aspect of the iliotibial tract, approximately a third of the way down

  □ Innervation: Superior gluteal nerve (L4 to S1)

  □ Other actions: Assists with internal rotation of the hip, assists with knee extension, and adds stability of the extended knee in standing and during ambulation

  □ Palpation site: Palpate inferiorly and slightly lateral to the anterior superior iliac spine

## Secondary Movers

- Gluteus medius
- Gluteus minimus

## Anti-Gravity

**Patient position:** Sidelying with the nontested limb resting in the anatomical position on the table top. The limb to be tested is positioned in approximately 45 degrees of hip flexion with the knee in extension. The foot should be resting on the table top.

**Stabilization:** The clinician stabilizes the pelvis.

- Grades 5/5 to +3/5: See Figure 7-41

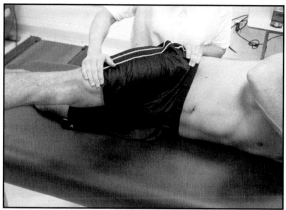

**Figure 7-41.** Resistance is applied on the lateral aspect of the thigh just proximal to the knee joint while the patient maintains 45 degrees of hip flexion.

PATIENT DIRECTIVE: *"Raise your leg up toward the ceiling and hold it. Do not let me push it down."*

- Grades 3/5 to +2/5: See Figure 7-42

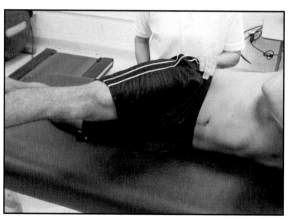

**Figure 7-42.** The patient abducts the hip through the maximal range of motion, maintaining 45 degrees of hip flexion without resistance.

MMT

## Gravity Minimized

**Patient position:** Long-sitting on a table with the arms behind the trunk for support, trunk leaning back to put the hips in approximately 45 degrees of flexion. The distal end of the tested limb is supported by the clinician's hand but should not interfere with or assist the movement.

**Stabilization:** Stabilization is achieved by the weight of the pelvis on the table top.

- Grades 2/5: See Figure 7-43

**Figure 7-43.** The paitent is able to abduct the lower extremity (to 30 degrees) while maintaining 45 degrees of hip flexion.

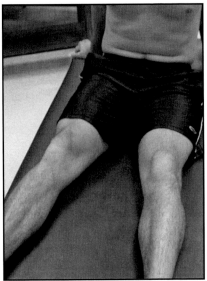

- Grades 1/5 to 0/5: See Figure 7-44

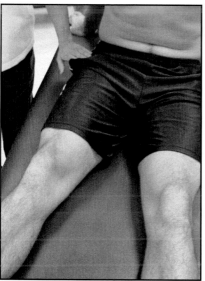

**Figure 7-44.** The tensor fascia latae is palpated inferiorly and slightly lateral to the anterior superior iliac spine as the patient attempts to abduct the hip.

**Points of interest:** Excessive tightness of the tensor facscia latae bilaterally may result in an anterior pelvis tilt and may contribute to genu valgum. Unilateral tightness of the tensor fascia latae may result in a lateral pelvic tilt.

## Adduction

### Active Range of Motion

- 0 degrees to 30 degrees

### Prime Movers

- Adductor magnus

  - ☐ Origin: Inferior ramus of the pubis and ischium and ischial tuberosity

  - ☐ Insertion: Linea aspera, medial supracondylar line, gluteal tuberosity, and adductor tubercle of the femur

  - ☐ Innervation: Obturator nerve (L2 to L3) and the tibial division of the sciatic nerve (L2 to L4)

  - ☐ Other actions: Assists with hip flexion/extension and hip internal/external rotation

  - ☐ Palpation site: Palpate along the middle to lower half of the medial aspect of the thigh

- Adductor longus

  - ☐ Origin: Anterior surface of the pubis in the angle between the crest and symphysis

  - ☐ Insertion: Middle third of the linea aspera of the femur

  - ☐ Innervation: Obturator nerve (L2 to L4)

  - ☐ Other actions: Slight hip flexion

  - ☐ Palpation site: Palpate just inferior to the pubic arch on the medial aspect of the thigh

- Adductor brevis

  - ☐ Origin: Inferior aspect of the pubis ramus

  - ☐ Insertion: Distal pectineal line and proximal portion of the linea aspera of the femur

  - ☐ Innervation: Obturator nerve (L2 to L4)

  - ☐ Other actions: Slight hip flexion

  - ☐ Palpation site: Too deep to palpate

- Pectineus
    - Origin: Superior pubic ramus
    - Insertion: Line from the lesser trochanter of the femur to the linea aspera
    - Innervation: Femoral nerve (L2 to L3) and the obturator nerve (L2 to L3)
    - Other actions: Hip flexion, slight internal rotation of the hip
    - Palpation site: Too deep to palpate
- Gracilis
    - Origin: Inferior aspect of the pubic ramus and symphysis
    - Insertion: Distal to the medial condyle of the tibia
    - Innervation: Obturator nerve (L2 to L3)
    - Other actions: Assists with knee flexion. Slight internal rotation of the tibia when the knee is in flexion
    - Palpation site: Palpate the tendon of the gracilis on the medial aspect of the knee

## Secondary Movers

- Obturator externus
- Inferior fibers of the gluteus maximus

## Anti-Gravity

**Patient position:** Sidelying with the tested limb resting on the table and the nontested limb supported by the clinician in a position of 25 degrees of abduction.

**Stabilization:** The pelvis is stabilized by the clinician against the table top.

MMT

• Grades 5/5 to +3/5: See Figure 7-45

**Figure 7-45**. Resistance is applied proximal to the knee joint on the medial aspect of the thigh into abduction.

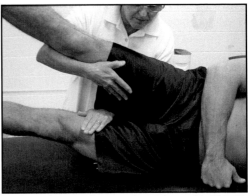

PATIENT DIRECTIVE: *"Lift your lower leg up so it meets the top leg and hold it. Do not let me push it down."*

• Grades 3/5 to +2/5: See Figure 7-46

**Figure 7-46**. The patient adducts the hip through the maximal range of motion without resistance.

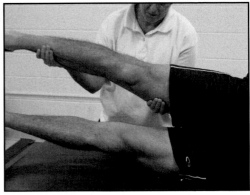

## Gravity Minimized

**Patient position:** Supine with the tested limb supported by the clinician in a slight amount of abduction and the nontested limb resting in 25 degrees of abduction.

**Stabilization:** Stabilization is achieved through the weight of the pelvis/trunk on the table top.

- Grades 2/5 to –2/5: See Figure 7-47

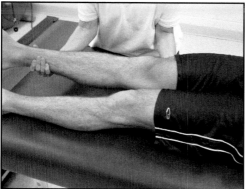

**Figure 7-47.** The patient adducts the hip through the maximal range of motion.

- Grades 1/5 to 0/5: See Figure 7-48

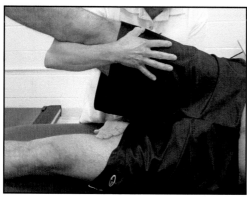

**Figure 7-48.** The adductor longus is palpated on the medial aspect of the thigh just inferior to the pubic arch, the adductor magnus is palpable along the medial aspect of the thigh (middle to lower portion), and the gracilis can be palpated along the medial aspect of the knee as the patient attempts to adduct the limb. (Shown: Palpating the adductor magnus.)

**Substitutions:** The patient may internally rotate the hip in an attempt to use the hip flexors to substitute for the hip adductors. The patient may externally rotate the hip in an attempt to substitute the hamstrings for the hip adductors during the movement.

**Points of interest:** It is not possible to isolate individual muscles during testing, so the adductors must be tested as a group. Depending on whether or not the femur is in flexion or extension, the adductors may assist during internal or external rotary movements of the hip.

MMT

# Internal (Medial) Rotation

## Active Range of Motion

- 0 degrees to 45 degrees (with the hip flexed)
- 0 degrees to 30 degrees (with the hip extended)

## Prime Movers

- Gluteus medius (anterior fibers)

    □ Origin: Outer surface of the ilium from the iliac crest and posterior gluteal line above to the anterior gluteal line below

    □ Insertion: Lateral surface of the greater trochanter

    □ Innervation: Superior gluteal nerve (L4 to S1)

    □ Other actions: Hip abduction

    □ Palpation site: Just proximal to the greater trochanter and laterally just distal to the iliac crest

- Gluteus minimus (anterior fibers)

    □ Origin: External surface of the ilium and inferior gluteal line

    □ Insertion: Anterior surface of the greater trochanter

    □ Innervation: Superior gluteal nerve (L4 to S1)

    □ Other actions: Hip abduction

    □ Palpation site: The gluteus minimus lies deep to the gluteus maximus and is not palpable

- Tensor fasciae latae

    □ Origin: Anterior aspect of the outer lip of the iliac crest and the anterior border of the ilium

    □ Insertion: Lateral aspect of the iliotibial tract, approximately two-thirds of the way down

- ☐ Innervation: Superior gluteal nerve (L4 to S1)

- ☐ Other actions: Hip flexion, abduction, and knee extension; it also adds stability to the extended knee when standing and during ambulation

- ☐ Palpation site: Palpate inferiorly and slightly lateral to the anterior superior iliac spine

## Secondary Movers

- Semitendinosus

- Semimembranosus

- Adductor magnus

- Adductor longus

## Anti-Gravity

**Patient position:** Sitting, with the knees flexed over the edge of a table.

**Stabilization:** The clinician stabilizes the distal thigh and the medial side of the knee joint.

- Grades 5/5 to +3/5: See Figure 7-49

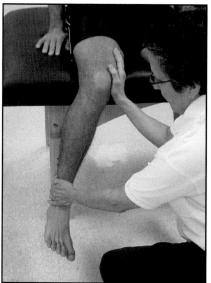

**Figure 7-49**. Resistance is applied to the lower leg just proximal to the lateral malleolus into external rotation.

PATIENT DIRECTIVE: *"Rotate your lower leg away from your other leg and hold it. Do not let me push it in."*

• Grades 3/5 to +2/5: See Figure 7-50

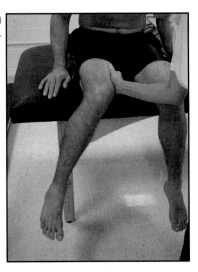

**Figure 7-50**. The patient internally rotates the tested leg through the maximal range of motion without resistance.

## Gravity Minimized

**Patient position:** Supine with the knees extended and the tested hip in slight external rotation.

**Stabilization:** The clinician stabilizes the pelvis against the table top.

• Grades 2/5 to –2/5: See Figure 7-51

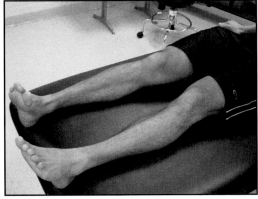

**Figure 7-51**. The patient internally rotates the hip through the available range of motion.

- Grades 1/5 to 0/5: See Figure 7-52

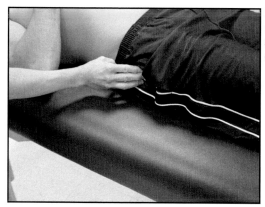

**Figure 7-52**. Only the anterior and middle fibers of the gluteus medius are palpable laterally below the crest of the ilium.

**Substitutions:** The patient may lift the pelvis off the table on the tested side, extend the knee/hip, or adduct the hip during testing.

MMT

# External (Lateral) Rotation

## Active Range of Motion

- 0 degrees to 45 degrees (with the hip flexed)
- 0 degrees to 30 degrees (with the hip extended)

### Prime Movers

- Obturator externus
  - □ Origin: External surface of the obturator membrane, inferior ramus of the pubis and ischium
  - □ Insertion: Trochanteric fossa of the femur
  - □ Innervation: Obturator nerve (L3 to L4)
  - □ Other actions: None
  - □ Palpation site: Too deep to palpate
- Obturator internus
  - □ Origin: Internal margin of the obturator foramen, ischial ramus, and obturator membrane
  - □ Insertion: Medial aspect of the greater trochanter of the femur
  - □ Innervation: Obturator nerve (L3 to L4)
  - □ Other actions: None
  - □ Palpation site: Too deep to palpate
- Piriformis
  - □ Origin: Anterior surface of the sacrum, gluteal surface of the ilium near the posterior inferior iliac spine, sacrotuberous ligament, capsule of the sacroiliac joint/border of the greater sciatic foramen
  - □ Insertion: Superior surface of the greater trochanter of the femur
  - □ Innervation: Sacral nerve (S1 to S2)
  - □ Other actions: None
  - □ Palpation site: Too deep to palpate

MMT

- Superior gemellus
  - □ Origin: Dorsal surface of the ischial spine
  - □ Insertion: Medial surface of the greater trochanter
  - □ Innervation: Obturator nerve/sacral plexus (L5 to S1)
  - □ Other actions: None
  - □ Palpation site: Too deep to palpate
- Inferior gemellus
  - □ Origin: Ischial tuberosity
  - □ Insertion: Medial surface of the greater trochanter of the femur, blending with the tendon of the obturator internus
  - □ Innervation: Obturator nerve/sacral plexus (L5 to S1)
  - □ Other actions: None
  - □ Palpation site: Too deep to palpate
- Quadratus femoris
  - □ Origin: Lateral aspect of the ischial tuberosity
  - □ Insertion: Intertrochanteric crest
  - □ Innervation: Sacral plexus (L5 to S1)
  - □ Other actions: None
  - □ Palpation site: Too deep to palpate

## Secondary Movers

- Sartorius
- Long head of the biceps femoris
- Posterior aspect of the gluteus medius
- Psoas major
- Adductor magnus
- Adductor longus
- Popliteus (with a fixed tibia)

MMT

## Anti-Gravity

**Patient position:** Sitting, with the knees flexed over the edge of a table.

**Stabilization:** The clinician stabilizes the distal thigh/knee joint on the lateral side.

- Grades 5/5 to +3/5: See Figure 7-53

**Figure 7-53.** Resistance is applied to the lower leg just proximal to the medial malleolus into internal rotation.

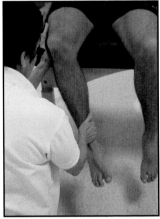

PATIENT DIRECTIVE: *"Rotate your lower leg toward your other leg and hold it. Do not let me push it out."*

- Grades 3/5 to +2/5: See Figure 7-54

**Figure 7-54.** The patient externally rotates the tested hip through the maximal range of motion without resistance.

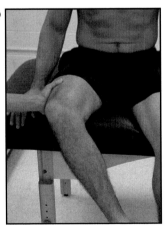

## Gravity Minimized

**Patient position:** Supine with the knees extended and the tested hip in slight internal rotation.

**Stabilization:** The clinician stabilizes the pelvis against the table top.

- Grades 2/5 to –2/5: See Figure 7-55

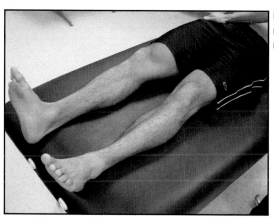

**Figure 7-55.** The patient externally rotates the hip through the maximal range of motion.

Because the external rotators are too deep to palpate (except for the gluteus maximus), a grade of 1/5 should be assigned if any contractile activity is observed. If the clinician is in doubt that the movement seen is a result of the lateral rotators contracting, a grade of 0/5 is appropriate.

**Substitutions:** In the anti-gravity position, the patient may lift the contracting buttock off the table, flex the knee, and abduct/adduct the hip during testing to substitute for hip external rotation.

**Points of interest:** The sciatic nerve runs between the lateral rotators of the femur and piriformis and may become entrapped or compressed by the piriformis, causing buttock and/or posterior thigh pain. These small muscles may be remembered in anatomical order from superior to inferior by the acronym "Piece Goods Often Go On Quilts" (Piriformis, Gemellus superior, Obturator internus, Gemellus inferior, Obturator externus, and Quadratus femoris).

MMT

# KNEE

## Flexion

### Active Range of Motion

- 0 degrees to 120 degrees (with the hip in extension)
- 0 degrees to 135 degrees (with the hip in flexion)

### Prime Movers

- Biceps femoris
  - □ Origin
    - o Long head: Ischial tuberosity and sacrotuberous ligament
    - o Short head: Linea aspera of the femur, lateral/proximal supracondylar line of the femur
  - □ Insertion
    - o Long and short heads: Head of the fibula and lateral tibial condyle
  - □ Innervation
    - o Long head: Tibial division of the sciatic nerve (L5 to S2)
    - o Short head: Peroneal division of the sciatic nerve (L5 to S2)
  - □ Other actions: Hip extension and external rotation of the tibia when the knee is flexed
  - □ Palpation site: Along the lateral/posterior thigh, immediately proximal to the knee joint
- Semitendinosus
  - □ Origin: Ischial tuberosity
  - □ Insertion: Proximal/medial shaft of the tibia; pes anserine

- ☐ Innervation: Tibial division of the sciatic nerve (L5 to S2)

- ☐ Other actions: Hip extension and internal rotation of the tibia when the knee is flexed

- ☐ Palpation site: Just proximal to the posterior knee joint line on the medial side

- Semimembranosus

  - ☐ Origin: Ischial tuberosity

  - ☐ Insertion: Posteromedial aspect of the medial tibial condyle

  - ☐ Innervation: Tibial division of the sciatic nerve (L5 to S2)

  - ☐ Other actions: Hip extension and internal rotation of the tibia when the knee is flexed

  - ☐ Palpation site: Just proximal to the posterior knee joint line on both sides of the semitendinosus tendon with the knee in slight flexion (between 0 degrees and 45 degrees)

## Secondary Movers

- Gracilis

- Tensor fasciae latae

- Sartorius

- Popliteus

- Gastrocnemius

- Plantaris

## Anti-Gravity

**Patient position:** Prone with the tested hip in neutral rotation and the knee flexed to approximately 45 degrees.

**Stabilization:** The clinician stabilizes the thigh against the table.

MMT

- Grades 5/5 to +3/5: See Figure 7-56

**Figure 7-56.** Resistance is applied just proximal to the posterior aspect of the ankle joint into knee extension.

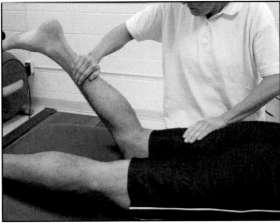

PATIENT DIRECTIVE: *"Bend your knee and hold it. Do not let me push it down."*

*\*To test the medial hamstrings (semitendinosus/semimembranosus), the tibia should be maintained in internal rotation. To test the lateral hamstring (biceps femoris), the tibia should be maintained in external rotation.*

- Grades 3/5 to +2/5: See Figure 7-57

**Figure 7-57.** The patient flexes the knee through the range of motion and is able to hold the end range position against gravity.

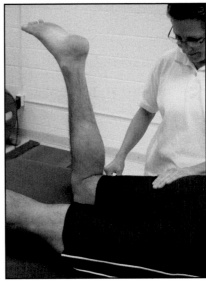

## Gravity Minimized

**Patient position:** Sidelying with the tested limb on top and either supported by the clinician or resting on a powder board. The lower limb is slightly flexed for stability.

**Stabilization:** The clinician stabilizes the thigh to prevent the hip from flexing during testing.

• Grades 2/5 to –2/5: See Figure 7-58

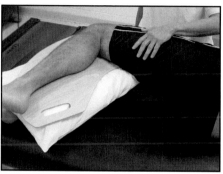

**Figure 7-58.** The patient flexes the knee through the maximal range of motion.

• Grades 1/5 to 0/5: See Figure 7-59

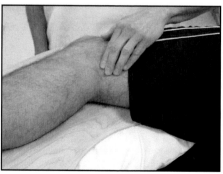

**Figure 7-59.** The tendon of the biceps femoris is visible and palpated along the posterior thigh just proximal to the posteriolateral aspect of the knee. The tendons of the semitendinosus and semimembranosus are visible and palpated just proximal to the posteromedial aspect of the knee joint as the patient attempts to flex the knee. (Shown: Palpating the biceps femoris.)

**Substitutions:** The hip may abduct/adduct or flex as the patient attempts to flex the knee because of the actions of the gracilis and sartorius. In addition, the gastrocnemius may cause plantarflexion of the ankle during testing.

*If the lateral hamstring is stronger than the medial hamstrings, the tibia will externally rotate during testing. If the medial hamstrings are stronger than the lateral hamstring, the tibia will internally rotate during testing.*

MMT

## Extension

### Active Range of Motion

- 120 degrees to 0 degrees (from knee flexion with the hip extended)
- 135 degrees to 0 degrees (from knee flexion with the hip flexed)

### Prime Movers

- Rectus femoris
  - □ Origin: Anterior inferior iliac spine and the superior rim of the acetabulum
  - □ Insertion: Tibial tuberosity via the patellar ligament
  - □ Innervation: Femoral nerve (L2 to L4)
  - □ Other actions: Hip flexion
  - □ Palpation site: Between the sartorius and tensor fascia latae of the proximal thigh
- Vastus intermedius
  - □ Origin: Upper two-thirds of the anterior and lateral shaft of the femur and the distal half of the linea aspera
  - □ Insertion: Tibial tuberosity via the patellar ligament
  - □ Innervation: Femoral nerve (L2 to L4)
  - □ Other actions: None
  - □ Palpation site: Too deep to palpate
- Vastus medialis
  - □ Origin: Medial lip of the linea aspera of the femur, distal intertrochanteric line, origin of the vastus medialis oblique, proximal supracondylar line, and tendon of the adductor magnus
  - □ Insertion: Tibial tuberosity via the patellar ligament
  - □ Innervation: Femoral nerve (L2 to L4)
  - □ Other actions: None
  - □ Palpation site: Medial aspect to the thigh, just proximal to the patella

MMT

- Vastus lateralis

    □ Origin: Lateral lip of the linea aspera of the femur, proximal aspect of the intertrochanteric line, inferior greater trochanter, lateral lip of the gluteal tuberosity

    □ Insertion: Tibial tuberosity via the patellar ligament

    □ Innervation: Femoral nerve (L2 to L4)

    □ Other actions: None

    □ Palpation site: Lateral aspect of the thigh

## Secondary Movers

- Tensor fasciae latae

## Anti-Gravity

**Patient position:** Sitting with both knees flexed to 90 degrees and hanging freely over the edge of a table.

**Stabilization:** The weight of the trunk and thigh provide stabilization for the lower leg.

- Grades 5/5 to +3/5: See Figure 7-60

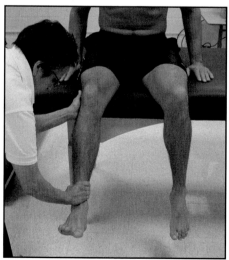

**Figure 7-60.** Resistance is applied just proximal to the ankle joint on the anterior aspect of the lower leg.

MMT

PATIENT DIRECTIVE: *"Straighten out your knee and hold it up. Do not let me push it down."*

- Grades 3/5 to +2/5: See Figure 7-61

**Figure 7-61**. The patient is able to extend the knee through the maximal range of motion and is able to hold the end range position without resistance.

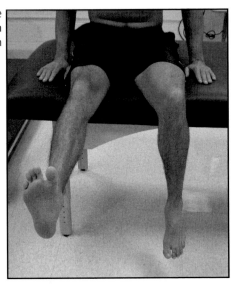

## Gravity Minimized

**Patient postion:** Sidelying with the tested limb on top resting on a powder board with the knee flexed to 90 degrees. The bottom knee should be slightly flexed for improved stability.

**Stabilization:** Stabilization is achieved through the weight of the lower limb, pelvis, and trunk lying against the table.

- Grades 2/5 to –2/5: See Figure 7-62

**Figure 7-62**. The patient extends the tested knee through the maximal range of motion.

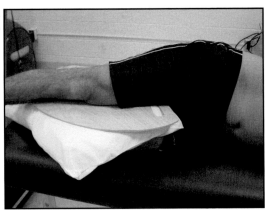

• Grades 1/5 to 0/5: See Figure 7-63

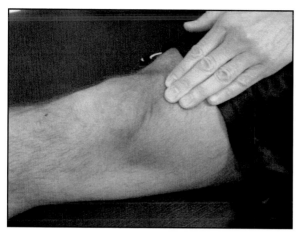

**Figure 7-63.** With the patient lying supine, the distal aspect of the quadriceps muscle group is palpated just proximal to the patella as the patient attempts to contract the anterior thigh.

**Substitutions:** The patient may attempt to internally rotate or extend the hip, allowing the knee to passively move into extension.

**Points of interest:** The rectus femoris is the only muscle in the quadriceps femoris group that crosses both the hip and knee joints. Its actions move the lower extremity forward while ambulating and extend the knee when performing a closed chain activity, such as jumping. Weakness of the quadriceps group impairs the ability to move sit to stand, ambulate uphill, or stair climb.

MMT

# ANKLE

## Dorsiflexion/Inversion

### Prime Movers

- Tibialis anterior

  □ Origin: Distal to the lateral tibial condyle, proximal/lateral half of the surface of the tibial shaft, and medial aspect of the fibula and the anterior interosseus membrane

  □ Insertion: Medial and plantar surface of the medial cuneiform bone and base of the first metatarsal

  □ Innervation: Deep peroneal nerve (L4 to S1)

  □ Other actions: None

  □ Palpation site: Along the lateral side of the tibia and as the tendon crosses the dorsum of the foot from the medial to lateral side

### Secondary Movers

- Peroneus tertius

- Extensor digitorum longus

- Extensor hallucis longus

### Anti-Gravity

**Patient position:** Sitting with the knee flexed over the edge of a table with the ankle/foot in a relaxed position.

*Alternate position: The patient may lie in supine with the ankle/foot hanging freely over the edge of a table.*

**Stabilization:** The thigh is stabilized against the table top while the clinician stabilizes the lower leg.

- Grades 5/5 to +3/5: See Figure 7-64

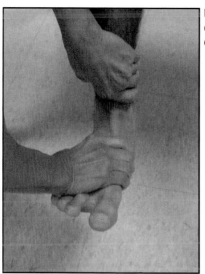

**Figure 7-64**. Resistance is applied to the medial/dorsal surface of the forefoot into plantarflexion and eversion.

PATIENT DIRECTIVE: *"Move your foot up toward your nose and in and hold it there. Do not let me push it down."*

- Grades 3/5 to +2/5: See Figure 7-65

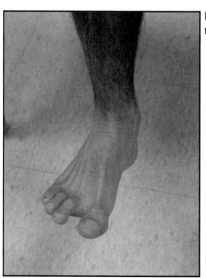

**Figure 7-65**. The patient dorsiflexes the ankle through the maximal range of motion without resistance.

## Gravity Minimized

**Patient position:** Sidelying with the tested limb/ankle on top resting on a powder board or smooth surface.

- Grades 2/5 to −2/5: See Figure 7-66

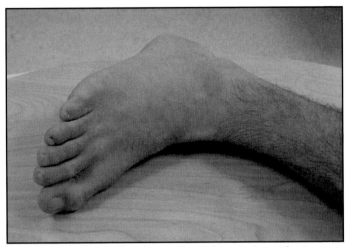

**Figure 7-66.** The patient dorsiflexes the ankle through the maximal range of motion.

- Grades 1/5 to 0/5: See Figure 7-67

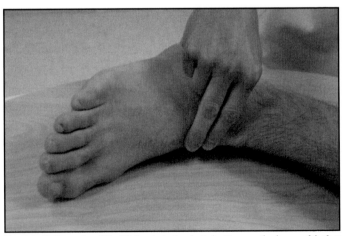

**Figure 7-67.** The tendon of the tibialis anterior is palpated as it crosses the dorsum of the foot as the patient attempts to dorsiflex the ankle.

**Substitutions:** The extensor digitorum longus and extensor hallucis longus may contract, causing toe extension. The tibialis posterior will cause inversion without dorsiflexion and the extensor digitorum longus will cause dorsiflexion with eversion.

# Plantarflexion

## Active Range of Motion

- 0 degrees to 45 degrees

## Prime Movers

- Gastrocnemius

  □ Origin

    o Medial head: Popliteal surface of the medial femoral condyle and capsule of the knee joint

    o Lateral head: Lateral surface of the lateral femoral condyle and capsule of the knee joint

  □ Insertion: Posterior surface of the calcaneus via the Achilles tendon

  □ Innervation: Tibial nerve (S1 to S2)

  □ Other actions: Flexion of the knee

  □ Palpation site: Immediately distal to the posterior knee joint line

- Plantaris

  □ Origin: Lateral supracondylar line of the femur

  □ Insertion: Medial aspect of the posterior part of the calcaneus via the Achilles' tendon

  □ Innervation: Tibial nerve (S1 to S2)

  □ Other actions: Slight knee flexion

  □ Palpation site: Too deep to palpate

- Soleus

  □ Origin: Head of the fibula, proximal third of the fibular shaft, soleal line, and mid-shaft of the posterior/medial border of the tibia

  □ Insertion: Medial side of the posterior surface of the calcaneus via the Achilles' tendon

  □ Innervation: Tibial nerve (S1 to S2)

  □ Other actions: None

  □ Palpation site: Bilaterally distal to the belly of the gastrocnemius

MMT

## Secondary Movers

- Tibialis posterior

- Peroneus longus

- Peroneus brevis

- Flexor digitorum longus

- Flexor hallucis longus

## Anti-Gravity

**Patient position:** Single-leg standing on the tested limb with the knee in maximal extension. The opposite foot should be off the floor and the patient should balance themselves with 1 to 2 fingers on a table top or counter top.

**Stabilization:** Provided with 1 to 2 fingers on a table top or counter top.

- Grades 5/5 to 3/5: See Figures 7-68 and 7-69

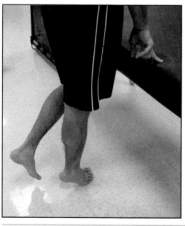

**Figure 7-68**. The patient easily completes at least 25 heel raises through the maximal range of motion with good form.

*Grade 4/5 is assigned if the patient is able to perform 10 to 24 heel raises through the maximal range of motion with good form and with no effort. Grade 3/5 is assigned if the patient is able to perform 1 to 9 heel raises through the maximal range of motion with good form and with no effort. The grade is dropped to the next lower level if patient is unable to complete the maximal range of motion on any given repetition.*

PATIENT DIRECTIVE: *"Stand on your right leg and push up onto your toes. Please repeat this as many times as you can until I tell you to stop."*

MMT

**Figure 7-69.** To test the soleus individually, the patient should stand on the tested limb with the knee in slight flexion.

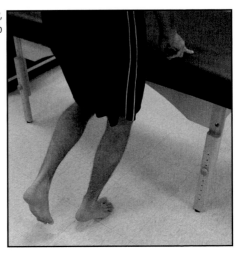

## Gravity Minimized

**Patient position:** Prone with the tested foot/ankle off the edge of a table.

**Stabilization:** Provided by the weight of the thigh/pelvis on the table top.

• Grade 2/5: See Figure 7-70A

• Grade +2/5: See Figure 7-70B

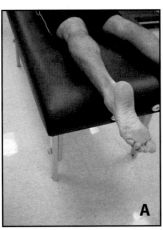 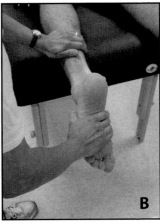

**Figures 7-70A and B.** The patient is able to plantarflex the ankle through the maximal range of motion.

*A grade of +2/5 is assigned if the patient can plantarflex through the maximal range of motion and hold it against maximal resistance. A grade of −2/5 is assigned if the patient completes partial range of motion without resistance.*

MMT

- Grades 1/5 to 0/5: See Figure 7-71

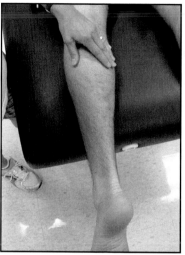

**Figure 7-71.** The gastrocnemius muscle is palpated at mid-calf with the thumb and fingers on either side of the muscle belly (above the soleus) and the soleus is palpated on the posterolateral surface of the distal calf as the patient attempts to plantarflex the ankle.
(Shown: Palpating the gastrocnemius.)

**Substitutions:** When standing, the patient may lean forward during testing, allowing the heel to passively raise off the floor. When lying in prone, substitution by the peroneus longus and brevis will cause the foot to move into eversion, and substitution by the tibialis posterior will cause the foot to invert. Substitution by the flexor hallucis longus and flexor digitorum longus will result in flexion of the toes and plantarflexion of the foot.

**Points of interest:** Although the gastrocnemius crosses both the knee and ankle joint, it can only act on the knee and ankle separately, not simultaneously. The word *soleus* is Latin for sole, which is a flat fish. This muscle lies deep to the gastrocnemius and is the stronger plantar flexor of the two. They are responsible for raising the heel during jumping or running.

MMT

# Inversion

## Active Range of Motion

- 0 degrees to 30 degrees

### Prime Movers

- Tibialis posterior

  ☐ Origin: Posterior surface of the shaft of the tibia, proximal two-thirds of the posterior aspect of the fibula, and the posterior interosseous membrane

  ☐ Insertion: Tuberosity of the navicular; plantar surface of the cuneiform bones; plantar surface of the basse of the second, third, and fourth metatarsals; the cuboid and sustentaculum tali

  ☐ Innervation: Tibial nerve (L4 to L5)

  ☐ Other actions: Plantarflexion of the ankle

  ☐ Palpation site: Between the medial malleolus and navicular

### Secondary Movers

- Tibialis anterior
- Flexor digitorum longus
- Flexor hallucis longus
- Soleus
- Extensor hallucis longus

### Anti-Gravity

**Patient position:** Sidelying with the tested foot and ankle over the edge of a table.

**Stabilization:** The lower limb is stabilized by the clinician against the table top.

MMT

- Grades 5/5 to +3/5: See Figure 7-72

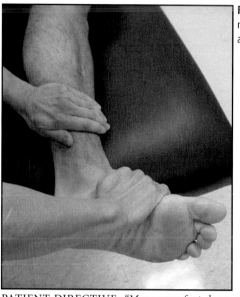

**Figure 7-72**. Resistance is applied to the medial border of the forefoot into eversion and dorsiflexion.

PATIENT DIRECTIVE: *"Move your foot down and in and hold it. Do not let me push it out."*

- Grades 3/5 to +2/5: See Figure 7-73

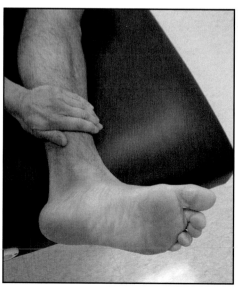

**Figure 7-73**. The patient is able to invert the foot through the maximal range of motion without resistance.

MMT

## Gravity Minimized

**Patient position:** Supine with the tested foot/ankle over the edge of a table.

**Stabilization:** The lower limb is stabilized by the clinician against the table top.

- Grades 2/5 to –2/5: See Figure 7-74

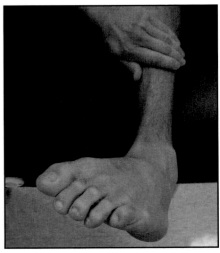

**Figure 7-74.** The patient is able to invert the foot through the maximal range of motion.

- Grades 1/5 to 0/5: See Figure 7-75

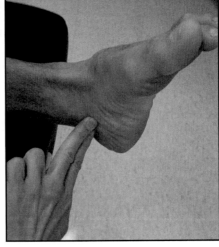

**Figure 7-75.** The posterior tibialis tendon is palpated as it crosses between the medial malleolus and navicular as the patient attempts to invert the ankle.

**Substitutions:** The tibialis anterior may cause dorsiflexion as the ankle inverts and the toe flexors may contribute to inversion and plantarflexion of the foot.

**Points of interest:** The tibialis posterior is the deepest of the posterior calf muscles whose tendons course around the medial malleolus (the others being the flexor digitorum longus and flexor hallucis longus), otherwise known as "Tom, Dick, and Harry." In addition to its primary actions, it is a major component of the longitudinal arch of the foot.

# Eversion

## Active Range of Motion

- 0 degrees to 25 degrees

## Prime Movers

- Peroneus longus

  - ☐ Origin: Lateral condyle of the tibia, head, and proximal two-thirds of the lateral surface of the fibula

  - ☐ Insertion: Lateral aspect of the first cuneiform bone and the base of the first metatarsal

  - ☐ Innervation: Superficial peroneal nerve (L5 to S1)

  - ☐ Other actions: Slight plantarflexion of the ankle

  - ☐ Palpation site: Just distal to the lateral malleolus as it runs to the plantar surface of the foot

- Peroneus brevis

  - ☐ Origin: Distal two-thirds of the lateral fibular shaft

  - ☐ Insertion: Tuberosity of the fifth metatarsal

  - ☐ Innervation: Superficial peroneal nerve (L5 to S1)

  - ☐ Other actions: Slight plantarflexion of the ankle

  - ☐ Palpation site: Just distal to the lateral malleolus as it runs anteriorly toward the fifth metatarsal

- Peroneus tertius

  - ☐ Origin: Lateral slip from the extensor digitorum longus

  - ☐ Insertion: Tuberosity of the fifth metatarsal

  - ☐ Innervation: Deep peroneal nerve (L5 to S1)

  - ☐ Other actions: Slight dorsiflexion of the ankle

  - ☐ Palpation site (if present): Laterally on the forefoot toward the fifth metatarsal

## Secondary Movers

- Extensor digitorum longus

## Anti-Gravity

**Patient position:** Sidelying with the tested foot and ankle over the edge of a table.

**Stabilization:** The lower limb is stabilized by the clinician against the table top.

· Grades 5/5 to +3/5: See Figure 7-76

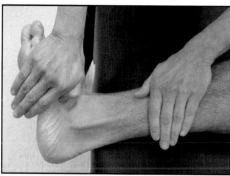

**Figure 7-76.** Resistance is applied to the lateral border of the forefoot into inversion and plantarflexion.

PATIENT DIRECTIVE: *"Move your foot up and out and hold it. Do not let me push it down."*

· Grades 3/5 to +2/5: See Figure 7-77

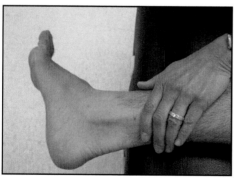

**Figure 7-77.** The patient is able to evert the foot through the maximal range of motion without resistance.

## Gravity Minimized

**Patient position:** Supine with the tested foot/ankle over the edge of a table.

**Stabilization:** The lower limb is stabilized by the clinician against the table top.

MMT

- Grades 2/5 to –2/5: See Figure 7-78

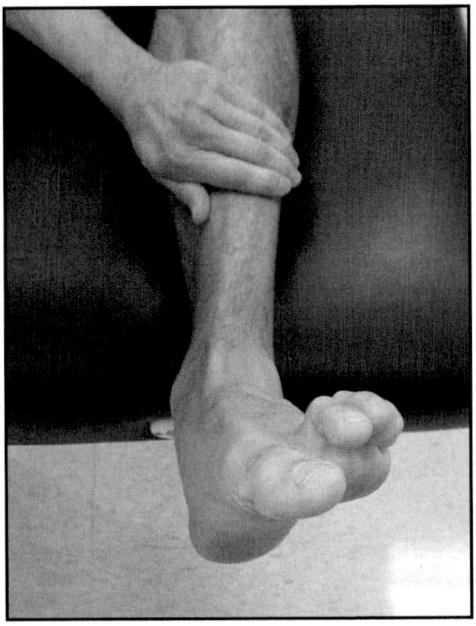

**Figure 7-78**. The patient is able to evert the foot through the maximal range of motion.

- Grades 1/5 to 0/5: See Figure 7-79

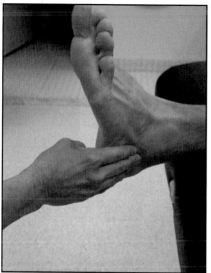

**Figure 7-79**. The tendons of the peroneus longus and brevis are palpated just distal to the lateral malleolus as the patient attempts to evert the ankle/foot.

**Substitutions:** Substitution by the extensor digitorum may cause the ankle to dorsiflex. The flexor digitorum may contract to cause eversion with some plantarflexion of the foot.

**Points of interest:** The actions of the ankle evertors are critical in keeping the ankle stable during activities taking place on uneven surfaces. The peroneus tertius acts to place the foot flat on the ground by raising the lateral border of the foot. This group may also be known as the "fibularis" longus, brevis, and tertius.

MMT

# GREAT TOE

*Note:* Because gravity is not a significant factor during testing of the toes, the format used for grading muscle strength deviates from the standard grading system applied to other muscle groups; half grades are not assigned.

## Flexion

### Active Range of Motion

- 0 degrees to 45 degrees (metatarsophalangeal [MTP] flexion)
- 0 degrees to 90 degrees (interphalangeal [IP] flexion)

### Prime Movers

- Flexor hallucis brevis
  - □ Origin
    - o Lateral head: Plantar surface of the cuboid and lateral cuneiform bone
    - o Medial head: Medial intermuscular septum and the tibialis posterior tendon
  - □ Insertion
    - o Lateral head: Proximal phalanx of the hallux (on both sides of the base) joining with the adductor hallucis
    - o Medial head: Proximal phalanx of the hallux (on both sides of the base) joining with the abductor hallucis
  - □ Innervation: Medial plantar nerve (S2)
  - □ Other actions: None
  - □ Palpation site: Along the medial arch of the foot, adjacent to the first metatarsal head
- Flexor hallucis longus
  - □ Origin: Distal two-thirds of the posterior aspect of the fibular shaft
  - □ Insertion: Base of the distal phalanx of the great toe

MMT

- ☐ Innervation: Tibial nerve (L5 to S2)

- ☐ Other actions: Slight plantarflexion of the ankle

- ☐ Palpation site: Palpate the tendon as it crosses the plantar surface of the proximal phalanx of the great toe

## Secondary Movers

- Adductor hallucis

- Abductor hallucis

### GRADES 5/5 (NORMAL), 4/5 (GOOD), 3/5 (FAIR), AND 2/5 (POOR)

**Patient position:** Sitting or supine with the tested knee in extension and the ankle and foot in neutral and resting on a table.

**Stabilization:** The foot is stabilized by the clinician.

- Grades 5/5 to 4/5: See Figure 7-80

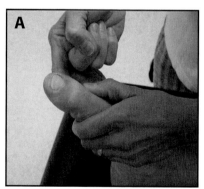 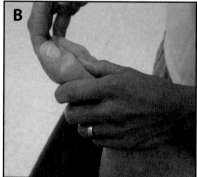

**Figure 7-80.** Resistance is applied on the plantar surfaces of the (A) proximal and (B) distal phalanx of the great toe to test the MTP and IP joints, respectively.

PATIENT DIRECTIVE: *"Curl your big toe over my finger and hold it. Do not let me straighten it out."*

MMT

- Grade 3/5: See Figure 7-81

**Figure 7-81**. The patient is able to flex the great toe through the maximal range of motion but is unable to maintain the position against resistance.

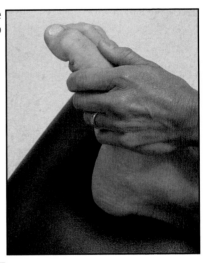

*Grade 2/5 is assigned for partial range of motion.*

## GRADES 1/5 (TRACE) AND 0/5 (ZERO)

- Grades 1/5 to 0/5: See Figure 7-82

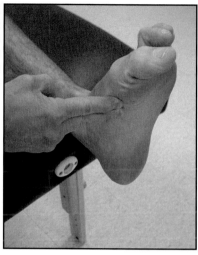

**Figure 7-82.** The flexor hallucis brevis is palpated along the medial arch of the foot, adjacent to the first metatarsal head and the flexor hallucis longus tendon is palpated as it crosses the plantar aspect of the proximal phalanx as the patient attempts to flex the great toe. (Shown: Palpating the flexor hallucis brevis.)

**Points of interest:** The flexor hallucis is active during walking and running by flexing the great toe to push off the ground.

## Extension

### Active Range of Motion

- 45 degrees to 0 degrees (MTP extension)
- 0 degrees to 90 degrees (MTP hyperextension)
- 90 degrees to 0 degrees (IP extension)

### Prime Movers

- Extensor hallucis brevis
  - ☐ Origin: Distal superolateral surface of the calcaneus
  - ☐ Insertion: Dorsal surface of the proximal phalanx
  - ☐ Innervation: Deep peroneal nerve (S1 to S2)
  - ☐ Other actions: None
  - ☐ Palpation site: Dorsolateral surface of the foot
- Extensor hallucis longus
  - ☐ Origin: Middle half of the medial aspect of the fibular shaft
  - ☐ Insertion: Base of the distal phalanx of the great toe
  - ☐ Innervation: Deep peroneal nerve (L5 to S1)
  - ☐ Other actions: Slight dorsiflexion of the ankle
  - ☐ Palpation site: Dorsum of the foot, lateral to the tibialis anterior tendon as it crosses the dorsal aspect of the first metatarsal

### Secondary Movers

- None

MMT

## GRADES 5/5 (NORMAL), 4/5 (GOOD), 3/5 (FAIR), AND 2/5 (POOR)

**Patient position:** Sitting or supine with both lower limbs extended and with the ankle and foot in neutral resting on a table.

**Stabilization:** The clinician stabilizes the foot and first metatarsal bone.

• Grades 5/5 to 4/5: See Figure 7-83

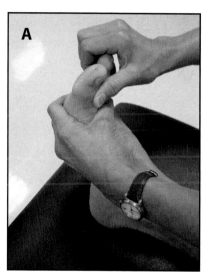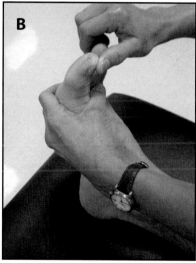

**Figure 7-83.** Resistance is applied to the dorsal surface of the (A) proximal and (B) distal phalanges of the great toe.

PATIENT DIRECTIVE: *"Straighten out your big toe and hold it. Do not let me push it down."*

- Grade 3/5: See Figure 7-84

**Figure 7-84.** The patient is able to actively extend the great toe through the maximal range of motion without resistance.

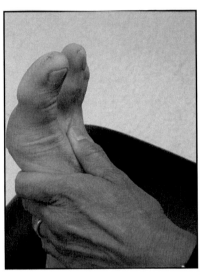

- Grade 2/5 is assigned for partial range of motion

## GRADES 1/5 (TRACE) AND 0/5 (ZERO)

**Patient position:** Sitting or supine with both lower limbs extended and with the ankle in neutral.

**Stabilization:** The clinician stabilizes the foot and first metatarsal bone. See Figure 7-85.

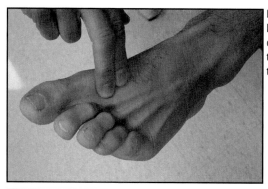

**Figure 7-85**. The extensor hallucis longus tendon is palpated on the dorsum of the foot lateral to the tibialis anterior tendon as it crosses the dorsum of the first metatarsal.

*Grade 1/5 is assigned if the tendon movement is observed or palpated as the patient attempts to extend the great toe.*

**Points of interest:** The strength of the extensor hallucis longus is assessed when suspecting L5 radiculopathy.

# TOES II TO V

## MTP Flexion

### Active Range of Motion

- 0 degrees to 40 degrees

### Prime Movers

- Lumbricals

    □ Origin: Medial and adjacent sides of the flexor digitorum longus tendon to each lateral digit

    □ Insertion: Medial aspect of the proximal phalanx and extensor hood of toes II to V

    □ Innervation: Lateral plantar nerve (L5 to S2)

    □ Other actions: Extension of the proximal interphalangeal (PIP)/distal interphalangeal (DIP) joints of toes II to V

    □ Palpation site: Too deep to palpate

### Secondary Movers

- Dorsal and plantar interossei
- Flexor digiti minimi brevis
- Flexor digitorum brevis
- Flexor digitorum longus

**GRADES 5/5 (NORMAL), 4/5 (GOOD), 3/5 (FAIR), AND 2/5 (POOR)**

**Patient position:** Sitting or supine with both limbs maximally extended and with the tested ankle/foot in neutral resting on a table.

**Stabilization:** The clinician stabilizes the lateral 4 metatarsal bones.

MMT

- Grades 5/5 and 4/5: See Figure 7-86

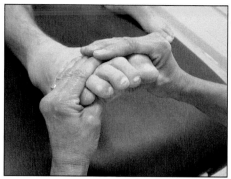

**Figure 7-86.** Resistance is applied to the plantar surface of the metatarsophalangeal joints of the 4 lateral toes into metatarsophalangeal extension.

PATIENT DIRECTIVE: *"Curl your toes over my fingers and hold it. Do not let me straighten them out."*

- Grade 3/5: See Figure 7-87

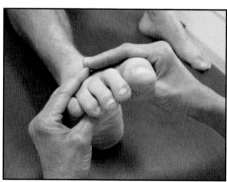

**Figure 7-87.** A grade of 3/5 is assigned if the patient is able to flex the metatarsophalangeal joints but is unable to hold them in position with any resistance. A grade of 2/5 is assigned if the patient can only move the toes through partial range of motion.

## GRADE 1/5 (TRACE) AND 0/5 (ZERO)

A grade of 1/5 is assigned if the clinician observes/palpates the contractile activity but no toe motion occurs.

**Points of interest:** Weakness of the lumbricals can result in hammer toes and loss of the transverse arch of the foot.

MMT

# DIP and PIP Flexion

## Active Range of Motion

- 0 degrees to 35 degrees (PIP)
- 0 degrees to 65 degrees (DIP)

### Prime Movers

- Flexor digitorum brevis
  - □ Origin: Medial process of the calcaneal tuberosity
  - □ Insertion: Tendon slips to the base of the middle phalanx of toes II to V
  - □ Innervation: Medial plantar nerve (S1 to S2)
  - □ Other actions: Flexion of the MTP joints of toes II to V
  - □ Palpation site: The tendons are palpable on the plantar surface of the proximal phalanx of toes II to V
- Flexor digitorum longus
  - □ Origin: Middle two-thirds of the posterior tibial shaft
  - □ Insertion: Base of the distal phalanx of toes II to V
  - □ Innervation: Tibial nerve (L5 to S2)
  - □ Other actions: Flexion of the MTP joints of toes II to V and slight plantarflexion of the ankle
  - □ Palpation site: The tendons are palpable on the plantar surface of each middle phalanx of toes II to V

### Secondary Movers

- Quadratus plantae

**GRADES 5/5 (NORMAL), 4/5 (GOOD), 3/5 (FAIR), AND 2/5 (POOR)**

**Patient position:** Sitting or supine with both lower extremities maximally extended and the ankle/foot in neutral resting on a table.

**Stabilization:** The clinician stabilizes the metatarsal bones of toes II to V.

MMT

- Grades 5/5 to 4/5: See Figure 7-88

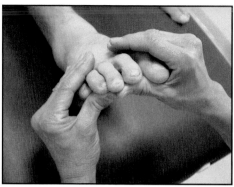

**Figure 7-88**. Resistance is applied under the plantar aspect of the proximal or distal phalanges, respectively, into extension.

PATIENT DIRECTIVE: *"Curl your toes over my fingers and hold it. Do not let me push them up."*

*A grade of 3/5 is assigned if the patient is able to complete the range of motion but is unable to do so with resistance. A grade of 2/5 is assigned if the patient only completes partial range of motion.*

## GRADES 1/5 (TRACE) AND 0/5 (ZERO)

- Grades 1/5 to 0/5: See Figure 7-89

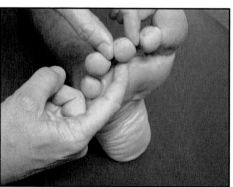

**Figure 7-89**. The tendons of the flexor digitorum longus are palpated on the plantar surface of the middle phalanx of toes II to V.

MMT

**Points of interest:** Weakness of the flexor digitorum longus may result in hyperpronation of the foot.

# DIP and PIP Extension

## Active Range of Motion

- 35 degrees to 0 degrees (PIP)
- 65 degrees to 0 degrees (DIP)

### Prime Movers

- Extensor digitorum brevis
  - Origin: Superolateral surface of the calcaneus
  - Insertion: Lateral sides of the tendons of the extensor digitorum longus
  - Innervation: Deep peroneal nerve (L5 to S1)
  - Other actions: Extension of the MTP joints of toes II to V
  - Palpation site: The muscle belly is palpable on the dorsolateral surface of the foot
- Extensor digitorum longus
  - Origin: Lateral condyle and lateral shaft of the tibia, proximal/anterior surface of the fibular shaft
  - Insertion: Dorsal surface of the middle/distal phalanges of digits II to V
  - Innervation: Deep peroneal nerve (L5 to S1)
  - Other actions: Extension of the MTP joints of toes II to V and slight dorsiflexion of the ankle joint
  - Palpation site: Dorsolateral surface of the foot to each of the 4 lateral digits

### Secondary Movers

- None

**GRADES 5/5 (NORMAL), 4/5 (GOOD), 3/5 (FAIR), AND 2/5 (POOR)**

**Patient position:** Sitting or supine with both lower extremities in maximal extension and the ankle/foot in neutral resting on a table.

**Stabilization:** The clinician stabilizes the metatarsal bones of toes II to V.

MMT

• Grades 5/5 to 4/5: See Figure 7-90

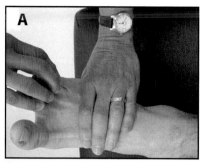 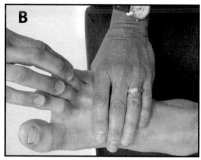

**Figure 7-90.** Resistance is applied to the dorsal surface of the (A) proximal and (B) distal phalanges into flexion to test PIP and DIP extension, respectively.

PATIENT DIRECTIVE: *"Straighten your toes and hold it. Do not let me push them down."*

*\*A grade of 3/5 is assigned if the patient is able to complete the range of motion but is unable to do so with resistance. A grade of 2/5 is assigned if the patient only completes partial range of motion.*

## GRADES 1/5 (TRACE) AND 0/5 (ZERO)

• Grades 1/5 and 0/5: See Figure 7-91

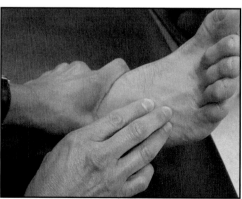

**Figure 7-91**. The tendons of the extensor digitorum longus are palpated as they cross the dorsolateral surface of the foot as they course to each of the lateral 4 toes.

MMT

# Appendices

# Appendix A: General Procedure for Goniometric Measurement

- The patient should be placed in a position closely correlating to the anatomical position in order to place the joints in a 0 starting position and to provide proper stabilization. It is important to attempt to position the patient in the same way each time the measurement is taken to ensure reliable results. The patient should be properly dressed in order to fully visualize the limb and allow free movement.

- It is important to explain the procedure to the patient and demonstrate the movement to ensure proper motion during measurement. Take a visual estimate to get an idea of the joint's range of motion.

- Make sure the proximal limb segment is stabilized to prevent substitution and inaccurate readings.

- Locate and if necessary mark the appropriate anatomic landmarks to help ensure proper alignment of the goniometer.

- Find the approximate axis of the joint being measured and place the fulcrum of the goniometer at this point.

- Align the stationary arm parallel to the longitudinal axis of the proximal portion of the limb segment and the movable arm parallel to the longitudinal axis of the distal limb segment, siting the appropriate landmarks. Keep in mind that it might be necessary to reverse the stationary arm to align it with the distal limb segment and align the movable arm with the proximal limb segment if the patient position or the goniometer itself does not allow for a proper reading. Proper alignment of the arms of the goniometer will ensure proper alignment of the fulcrum.

- Do not press the goniometer against the limb as this might distort the reading. Hold the arms with the thumb and first 2 fingers in order to clearly see the readings.

- Take the first reading at the beginning of the motion. Remove the goniometer. Allow the motion to occur (either actively or passively) and realign the goniometer at the end of the motion. Do not move the stationary arm that is aligned against the proximal body segment.

- If the patient has no limitations and is in the recommended testing position, assume the starting point is 0 degrees. The end point of the motion is recorded in a positive number away from 0. If there is an impairment and the movement does not start at 0, record the amount of limitation in degrees.

# Appendix B: Commonly Used Terms in Goniometry

**abduction:** Motion at a joint so that the distal segment is moved laterally away from the midline of the body.

**adduction:** Motion at a joint so that the distal segment is moved medially toward the midline of the body.

**axis of rotation:** A line at right angles to the plane in which adjacent limb segments move and about which all moving parts of the segments rotate in a circular path. Otherwise known as the "fulcrum," this is the point where both arms of the goniometer meet on the body of the protractor. It is identifiable by the rivet or tension knob connecting the 2 arms together. The axis of the goniometer should coincide with the axis of the joint being tested.

**deviation:** Moving away from a starting position; frequently to denote abduction or adduction relative to the midline or rotation from a starting point.

**dorsiflexion:** Flexing or bending of the foot toward the leg so that the angle between the dorsum of the foot and the leg is decreased.

**eversion:** Turning outward; turning the sole of the foot so it faces laterally.

**extension:** Movement of a joint so the 2 adjacent segments are moved apart and the joint angle is increased.

**flexion:** Movement of a joint so the 2 adjacent segments approach each other and the joint angle is decreased.

**fluid goniometer:** Consists of a 360-degree scale in a flat, fluid-filled circular tube that contains a small air bubble. The device is attached to or placed onto the limb or body part, and as the limb/body part moves, the scale rotates and the bubble remains stationary. The range of motion is read at the point the scale stops moving.

**frontal or coronal planes:** A vertical plane at right angles to the sagittal plane, dividing the body into ventral and dorsal halves.

**goniometer:** An instrument used to measure the joint movement and joint angles of the body.

**goniometry:** Derived from the Greek words "gonia," meaning angle, and "metron," meaning measure. The measurement of angles of the human body.

**horizontal or transverse plane:** Any plane through the body that divides the body into upper and lower halves.

**inversion:** Turning inward; turning the sole of the foot so it faces medially.

**lateral (external) rotation:** The rotation of a joint segment in the transverse plane around a vertical or longitudinal axis away from the midline of the body or toward the posterior surface of the body.

**longitudinal axis:** A line passing through a bone or segment, around which the parts are symmetrically arranged and lying in both the frontal and sagittal planes.

**medial (internal) rotation:** The rotation of a joint segment in the transverse plane around a vertical or longitudinal axis toward the midline of the body or toward the anterior surface of the body.

**moving arm:** The arm of the goniometer that is movable and is aligned with the segment that is distal to the joint being measured.

**opposition:** Moving the thumb away from the palm in a direction perpendicular to the plane of the hand allowing the thumb to touch the pad of the fifth digit.

**plantarflexion:** Flexing or bending of the foot in the direction of the sole so that the angle between the dorsum of the foot and leg is increased.

**pronation:** Rotating of the forearm so the palm of the hand is down or posterior in the anatomical position.

**rotation:** The turning or moving of a part around a fixed axis in a curved path.

**sagittal plane:** The vertical, anterior-posterior plane through the longitudinal axis of the trunk, dividing the body into right and left halves.

**stationary arm:** The arm of the goniometer that is fixed and aligned in parallel with the longitudinal axis of the segment proximal to the joint being measured.

**substitution:** A movement performed by the patient in an attempt to avoid pain caused by testing or to increase the joint range of motion.

**supination:** Rotating the forearm so the palm of the hand is up or anterior in the anatomical position.

**universal goniometer:** A plastic or metal device that consists of a protractor connected to 2 arms, 1 of which is attached to the body by a rivet. This is the most common type of goniometer used in the clinical setting.

# Appendix C: Normal Range of Motion Values in Adults

| Joint | AAOS | AMA | Boone & Azen | Daniels & Worthingham | Hoppenfeld |
|---|---|---|---|---|---|
| *Shoulder* | | | | | |
| Flexion | 180 | 180 | 167 | 90 | 90 |
| Extension | 60 | 50 | 62 | 50 | 45 |
| Abduction | 180 | 160 | 184 | 90 | 180 |
| Internal rotation | 70 | 90 | 69 | 90 | 55 |
| External rotation | 90 | 90 | 104 | 90 | 45 |
| Horizontal abduction | 45 | ----- | 45 | ----- | ----- |
| Horizontal adduction | 135 | 30 | 140 | ----- | ----- |
| *Elbow* | | | | | |
| Flexion | 150 | 135 | 143 | 160 | 150 |
| *Radioulnar* | | | | | |
| Pronation | 80 | 90 | 76 | 90 | 90 |
| Supination | 80 | 90 | 82 | 90 | 90 |
| *Wrist* | | | | | |
| Flexion | 80 | 50 | 76 | 90 | 80 |
| Extension | 70 | 60 | 75 | 70 | 70 |
| Radial deviation | 20 | 20 | 22 | 25 | 20 |
| Ulnar deviation | 30 | 30 | 36 | 65 | 30 |
| *Thumb—CMC* | | | | | |
| Abduction | 70 | 50 | ----- | 50 | 70 |
| Flexion | 15 | ----- | ----- | ----- | ----- |
| Extension | 20 | ----- | ----- | ----- | ----- |
| Opposition | Thumb tip to tip of 5th digit | 50 | ----- | Thumb tip to tip of 5th digit | Thumb tip to tip of 5th digit |
| *Thumb—MCP* | | | | | |
| Flexion | 50 | 60 | ----- | 70 | 50 |
| *Thumb—IP* | | | | | |
| Flexion | 80 | 80 | ----- | 90 | 90 |
| *Digits II-V—MCP* | | | | | |
| Flexion | 90 | 90 | ----- | 90 | 90 |
| Extension | 45 | 20 | ----- | 30 | 45 |
| Abduction | ----- | ----- | ----- | 25 | 20 |
| *Digits II-V—PIP* | | | | | |
| Flexion | 100 | 100 | ----- | 120 | 100 |
| *Digits II-V—DIP* | | | | | |
| Flexion | 90 | 100 | ----- | 80 | 90 |
| Extension | ----- | ----- | ----- | ----- | 10 |

| Joint | Kapanji | Gerhardt & Russe | AOA | Dorinson & Wagner | Kendall, Kendall, & Wadsworth |
|---|---|---|---|---|---|
| **Shoulder** | | | | | |
| Flexion | 180 | 170 | ----- | 180 | 180 |
| Extension | 50 | 50 | ----- | 45 | 45 |
| Abduction | 180 | 170 | ----- | 180 | 180 |
| Internal rotation | 95 | 80 | ----- | 90 | 70 |
| External rotation | 80 | 90 | ----- | 90 | 90 |
| Horizontal abduction | ----- | 30 | ----- | ----- | ----- |
| Horizontal adduction | ----- | 135 | ----- | ----- | ----- |
| **Elbow** | | | | | |
| Flexion | 145 | 150 | 146 | 150 | 145 |
| **Radioulnar** | | | | | |
| Pronation | 85 | 80 | 71 | 80 | 90 |
| Supination | 90 | 90 | 84 | 70 | 90 |
| **Wrist** | | | | | |
| Flexion | 85 | 60 | 73 | 80 | 80 |
| Extension | 85 | 50 | 71 | 55 | 70 |
| Radial deviation | 15 | 20 | 19 | 20 | 20 |
| Ulnar deviation | ----- | 30 | 33 | 40 | 35 |
| **Thumb—CMC** | | | | | |
| Abduction | ----- | ----- | ----- | 80 | ----- |
| Flexion | ----- | ----- | ----- | 50 | ----- |
| Extension | ----- | ----- | ----- | 50 | ----- |
| Opposition | ----- | ----- | ----- | Thumb tip to tip of 5th digit | ----- |
| **Thumb—MCP** | | | | | |
| Flexion | ----- | ----- | ----- | 80 | ----- |
| **Thumb—IP** | | | | | |
| Flexion | ----- | ----- | ----- | 90 | ----- |
| **Digits II-V—MCP** | | | | | |
| Flexion | ----- | ----- | ----- | ----- | ----- |
| Extension | ----- | ----- | ----- | ----- | ----- |
| Abduction | ----- | ----- | ----- | ----- | ----- |
| **Digits II-V—PIP** | | | | | |
| Flexion | ----- | ----- | ----- | 100 | ----- |
| **Digits II-V—DIP** | | | | | |
| Flexion | ----- | ----- | ----- | 80 | ----- |
| Extension | ----- | ----- | ----- | ----- | ----- |

| Joint | AAOS | AMA | Boone & Azen | Daniels & Worthingham | Hoppenfeld |
|---|---|---|---|---|---|
| *Hip* | | | | | |
| Flexion | 120 | 100 | 122 | 125 | 135 |
| Extension | 30 | 30 | 10 | 15 | 30 |
| Abduction | 45 | 45 | 46 | 45 | 50 |
| Adduction | 30 | 30 | 27 | 0 | 30 |
| Internal rotation | 45 | 40 | 47 | 45 | 35 |
| External rotation | 45 | 50 | 47 | 45 | 45 |
| *Knee* | | | | | |
| Flexion | 135 | 150 | 143 | 130 | 135 |
| *Ankle* | | | | | |
| Dorsiflexion | 20 | 20 | 13 | 90 | 90 |
| Plantarflexion | 50 | 40 | 56 | 90 | 90 |
| *Subtalar Joint* | | | | | |
| Inversion | 35 | 30 | 37 | ----- | 5 |
| Eversion | 15 | 20 | 26 | ----- | 5 |
| *Transverse Tarsal* | | | | | |
| Inversion | 20 | 30 | ----- | ----- | 20 |
| Eversion | 10 | 20 | ----- | ----- | 10 |
| *First Toe—MTP* | | | | | |
| Flexion | 45 | 30 | ----- | ----- | 45 |
| Extension | 70 | 50 | ----- | ----- | 90 |
| *First Toe—IP* | | | | | |
| Flexion | 90 | 30 | ----- | ----- | ----- |
| *Toes II-V—MTP* | | | | | |
| Flexion | 40 | 30 | ----- | 35 | ----- |
| Extension | 40 | 50 | ----- | ----- | ----- |
| *Toes II-V—PIP* | | | | | |
| Flexion | 35 | 30 | ----- | 90 | ----- |
| *Toes II-V—DIP* | | | | | |
| Flexion | ----- | ----- | ----- | ----- | ----- |

| Joint | Kapanji | Gerhardt & Russe | AOA | Dorinson & Wagner | Kendall, Kendall, & Wadsworth |
|---|---|---|---|---|---|
| **Hip** | | | | | |
| Flexion | 120 | 125 | ----- | ----- | 125 |
| Extension | 30 | 15 | ----- | ----- | 10 |
| Abduction | 30 | 45 | ----- | ----- | 45 |
| Adduction | 30 | 15 | ----- | ----- | ----- |
| Internal rotation | 30 | 45 | ----- | ----- | ----- |
| External rotation | 60 | 45 | ----- | ----- | ----- |
| **Knee** | | | | | |
| Flexion | 160 | 130 | 134 | ----- | 140 |
| **Ankle** | | | | | |
| Dorsiflexion | 30 | 20 | 18 | ----- | 20 |
| Plantarflexion | 50 | 45 | 48 | ----- | 45 |
| **Subtalar Joint** | | | | | |
| Inversion | 52 | 40 | 5 | ----- | ----- |
| Eversion | 30 | 20 | 5 | ----- | ----- |
| **Transverse Tarsal** | | | | | |
| Inversion | ----- | ----- | ----- | 50 | ----- |
| Eversion | ----- | ----- | ----- | 20 | ----- |
| **First Toe—MTP** | | | | | |
| Flexion | ----- | ----- | ----- | ----- | 30 |
| Extension | ----- | ----- | ----- | ----- | 40 |
| **First Toe—IP** | | | | | |
| Flexion | ----- | ----- | ----- | ----- | ----- |
| **Toes II-V—MTP** | | | | | |
| Flexion | ----- | ----- | ----- | ----- | ----- |
| Extension | ----- | ----- | ----- | ----- | ----- |
| **Toes II-V—PIP** | | | | | |
| Flexion | ----- | ----- | ----- | ----- | ----- |
| **Toes II-V—DIP** | | | | | |
| Flexion | ----- | ----- | ----- | ----- | ----- |

# Appendix D: Anatomical Zero

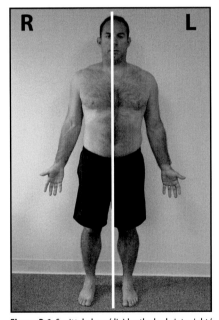

**Figure D-1**. Sagittal plane (divides the body into right/left).

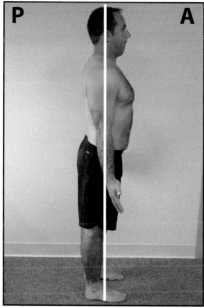

**Figure D-2**. Frontal plane (divides the body into anterior/posterior).

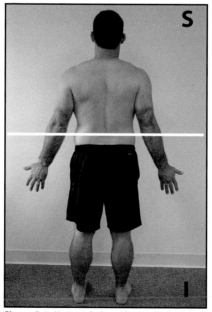

**Figure D-3**. Horizontal plane (divides the body into superior/inferior).

# Appendix E: Capsular Patterns

The Cervical Spine—lateral flexion = rotation/extension
The Scapulothoracic Joint—none
The Shoulder (Glenohumeral Joint)—external rotation > abduction > internal rotation
The Elbow (Humeroulnar and Humeroradial Joints)—flexion > extension
The Forearm (Radioulnar Joint)—pronation = supination
The Wrist (Radiocarpal and Intercarpal Joints)—equal restriction of all motions
The Fingers–Digits II to V (Metacarpophalangeal Joints)—flexion > extension
The Fingers–Digits II to V (Proximal Interphalangeal Joints)—flexion > extension
The Fingers–Digits II to V (Distal Interphalangeal Joints)—flexion > extension
The Thumb (Carpometacarpal Joint)—abduction > extension
The Thumb (Metacarpophalangeal Joint)—flexion > extension
The Thumb (Interphalangeal Joint)—flexion > extension
The Thoracolumbar Spine—lateral flexion = rotation/extension
The Hip—internal/external rotation > abduction > flexion > extension > adduction
The Knee (Tibiofemoral Joint)—flexion > extension
The Ankle—plantarflexion > dorsiflexion
The Subtalar Joint (Hindfoot)—none
The Transverse Tarsal Joint (Midfoot)—none
The First Toe (Metatarsophalangeal Joint)—extension > flexion
The First Toe (Interphalangeal Joint)—flexion > extension
Toes II to V (Metatarsophalangeal Joints)—flexion > extension
Toes II to V (Proximal Interphalangeal Joints)—flexion > extension
Toes II to V (Distal Interphalangeal Joints)—flexion > extension
The Temporomandibular Joint—restriction in the ability to open the mouth

# Appendix F: General Procedure for Manual Muscle Testing

- The patient should be positioned in a manner that ensures accurate testing and addresses comfort. The test position may need to be modified occasionally to minimize stress on other parts of the body.

- The patient should be positioned so that support is provided to the body as a whole so that the patient can focus on the body part being tested.

- The body part being tested should initially be placed in an anti-gravity position. If the muscles are too weak to function against gravity, the body part should be placed in a position in which gravity is minimized.

- The proximal aspect of the tested body part should be stabilized to decrease the compensatory action of other muscles that are not being tested.

- Resistance given during testing should be directly opposite to the "line of pull" of the muscles being tested.

- Resistance should be gradual and uniform, not sudden or "jerky." A long lever arm should be used unless contraindicated.

- Both sides of the body should be tested when appropriate to provide a comparison. This is especially important if there is a known injury/pathology of the tested side.

# Appendix G: Commonly Used Terms in Manual Muscle Testing

**active resisted test:** A muscle test in which the examiner gradually increases the amount of manual resistance until it reaches the maximal level the patient can tolerate and the movement stops. This type of testing is used infrequently because of the level of skill required to perform it accurately.

**available range of motion:** The full range of motion for that patient at the time of testing. Although it may not be normal, muscle grading is assigned within this range.

**break test:** A muscle test that is used to determine the maximal effort given by the patient when manual resistance is applied to the body part after it is placed at the end range position by the examiner. The patient is asked to "hold" the body part at the end of the available range of motion and not allow the examiner to "break" the hold with manual resistance. It is the most commonly used manual muscle testing procedure.

**grading:** The assignment of a word or numerical value based on an examiner's assessment of the strength or weakness of a muscle or muscle group. Grading values range from zero (0) to normal (5); 0 denotes no muscle activity and 5 denotes normal activity, which is considered the best possible effort by the patient to the test.

**resistance:** The external force that opposes the test movement.

**stabilization:** The holding steady or holding down of a body part to ensure an accurate test of a muscle or muscle group.

**substitution:** A movement that results from 1 or more muscles attempting to compensate for the lack of strength in a muscle group or group of muscles.

**test movement:** The movement of a body part in a specified direction through a specific arc of motion.

**test position:** The position in which the body part is placed by the examiner and held by the patient.

**weakness:** Loss of movement of a body part as a result of a muscle not contracting sufficiently to move the body part through partial or full range of motion.

# Appendix H: Factors That May Cause Inaccurate Muscle Testing

- The patient becomes distracted during testing.

- The patient experiences pain during testing.

- The patient is positioned improperly.

- The body part being tested is not adequately stabilized.

- Inability of the patient to understand the test requirements/commands as a result of poor comprehension or cultural and language barriers.

- The patient does not have the coordination to perform the test adequately.

- Inadequate understanding of basic anatomy/kinesiology by the clinician.

- Poor awareness of basic substitution patterns by the clinician.

- "Overgrading" or "undergrading" a muscle as a result of clinician inexperience.

- Inconsistency in timing, pressure, and positioning by the clinician.

- The use of gloves by the clinician may alter the ability to palpate a muscle contraction accurately.

- External devices or equipment in the environment may limit the clinician's ability to adequately test a body part.

# Appendix I: Precautions and Contraindications for Manual Muscle Testing

## Precautions

. Recent abdominal surgery

. Recent neurosurgery

. Recent eye injury

. Conditions in which fatigue may cause harm or an increase in symptoms (such as with chronic obstructive pulmonary disease, poliomyelitis, multiple sclerosis, Parkinson's disease, myasthenia gravis, intermittent claudication, malignancy)

. History of aneurysm

. Hypertension

. History of myocardial infarction or angina pectoris

. Cardiopulmonary disease

. Osteoporosis

. Hemophilia

. A recently healed fracture

. If the patient is taking pain medication or muscle relaxants as it may affect the patient's ability to respond appropriately

. After prolonged immobilization

## Contraindications

- Localized inflammation of the area being tested
- Inflammatory neuromuscular diseases (such as Guillain-Barré syndrome, polymyositis, and dermatomyositis)
- Severe cardiac disease
- Severe respiratory disease
- Presence of pain
- Risk of venous thromboembolism
- Subluxation/dislocation of a joint or unhealed fracture
- Myositis ossificans or ectopic ossification

Adapted from Clarkson HM. *Musculoskeletal assessment. Joint range of motion, muscle testing and function: a research-based practical guide.* 4th ed. Lippincott, Williams & Wilkins; 2021.

# Appendix J: Sample Goniometers, Smartphone Goniometer Application, and Other Tools for Muscle Testing

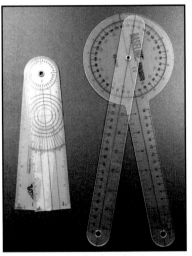

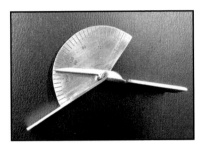

**Figure J-2**. Sample of a smaller goniometer commonly used for fingers and toes.

**Figure J-1**. Samples of traditional goniometers.

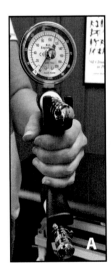

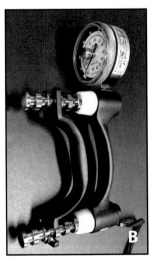

**Figure J-3**. Sample of a hand dynamometer used to measure grip strength.

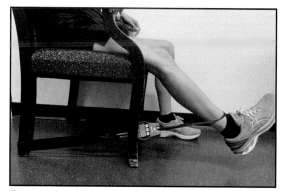

**Figure J-4**. Sample of a crane scale that can be used for a more precise measurement of muscle strength.

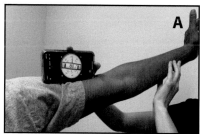

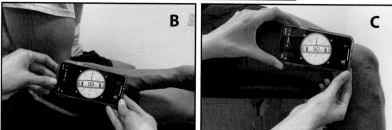

**Figure J-5**. Alternative methods of measurement with the use of a smartphone application may be used in place of a traditional goniometer. The reliability and validity of smartphone goniometers is relatively new and is currently being researched for clinical application.

# Bibliography

Abrahamson E, Langston J. *Muscle Testing—A Concise Manual.* Handspring Publishing; 2019.

American Academy of Orthopaedic Surgeons. *Joint Motion: Method of Measuring and Recording.* Author; 1965.

American Orthopaedic Association. *The Manual of Orthopaedic Surgery.* Author; 1972.

Amundsen LR, ed. *Muscle Strength Testing: Instrumented and Non-Instrumented Systems.* Churchill Livingstone; 1990.

Avers D, Brown M. *Daniels and Worthingham's Muscle Testing: Techniques of Manual Examination and Performance Testing.* 10th ed. Elsevier; 2019.

Basmajian JV, De Luca CJ. *Muscles Alive: Their Functions Revealed by Electromyography.* Williams & Wilkins; 1985.

Beasley WC. Quantitative muscle testing: principles and applications to research and clinical services. *Arch Phys Med Rehabil.* 1961;42:398-425.

Bernier J. *Quick Reference Dictionary for Athletic Training.* 2nd ed. SLACK Incorporated; 2005.

Bohannon RW. Internal consistency of manual muscle testing scores. *Percept Mot Skills.* 1997;85:736-738.

Bohannon RW. Make tests and break tests of elbow flexor muscle strength. *Phys Ther.* 1988;68:193-194.

Bohannon RW. Manual muscle testing: Does it meet the standards of an adequate screening test? *Clin Rehabil.* 2005;19:662-667.

Boone DC, Azen SP. Normal range of motion of joints in male subjects. *J Bone Joint Surg.* 1979;61:756-759.

Clark WA. A system of joint measurement. *J Orthop Surg.* 1920;2:687-700.

Clarkson HM. *Musculoskeletal Assessment. Joint Range of Motion, Muscle Testing and Function: A Research-Based Practical Guide.* 4th ed. Lippincott, Williams & Wilkins; 2021.

Cole JH, Furness AL, Twomey LT. *Muscles in action. An approach to manual muscle testing.* Churchill Livingstone; 1988.

Cuthbert SC, Goodheart GJ. On the reliability and validity of manual muscle testing: a literature review. *Chiropr Osteopat.* 2007;15.

Cutter NC, Kevorkian CG, eds. *Handbook of Manual Muscle Testing.* McGraw-Hill; 1999.

Daniels L, Worthingham C. *Manual Muscle Testing: Techniques of Manual Examination.* 3rd ed. WB Saunders; 1972.

Donatelli RA, Wooden MJ. *Orthopedic Physical Therapy.* 4th ed. Churchill Livingstone; 2010.

Dorinson SM, Wagner ML. An exact technique for clinically measuring and recording joint motion. *Arch Phys Med Rehabil.* 1948;29:468-475.

Durfee WK, Iaizzo PA. *Rehabilitation and Muscle Testing: Encyclopedia of Medical Devices and Instrumentation.* 2nd ed. John Wiley & Sons; 2006.

Dutton M. *Dutton's Orthopaedic Examination, Evaluation, and Intervention.* 5th ed. McGraw-Hill; 2020.

Elveru RA, Rothstein JM, Lamb RL, Riddle DL. Methods for taking subtalar joint measurements: a clinical report. *Phys Ther.* 1988;68:678-682.

Evans RC. *Illustrated Orthopedic Physical Assessment.* 3rd ed. Mosby; 2009.

Eyadah AA, Ivanova MK. Methods for measurement of tibial torsion. *J Kuwait Med Assoc.* 2001;33(1):3-6.

Fitzgerald GK, Wynveen KJ, Rheault W, et al. Objective assessment with establishment of normal values for lumbar spinal range of motion. *Phys Ther.* 1983;63(11):1776-1781.

Gerhardt JJ, Cocchiarella L, Lea RD. *The Practical Guide to Range of Motion Assessment.* American Medical Association Press; 2002.

Gerhardt JJ, Russe OA. *International SFTR Method of Measuring and Recording Joint Motion.* Hans Huber; 1975.

Greene WB, Heckman JD. (eds). *The Clinical Measurement of Joint Motion.* American Academy of Orthopaedic Surgeons; 1994.

Griffin LY. *Essentials of Musculoskeletal Care.* 3rd ed. American Academy of Orthopaedic Surgeons; 2005.

Hansen JT. *Netter's Clinical Anatomy.* 2nd ed. Saunders; 2010.

Hellebrandt FA, Duvall E, Moore ML. The measurement of joint motion. Reliability of goniometry. *Phys Ther Rev.* 1949;29(Pt 3):302.

Higbie EJ, Seidel-Cobb D, Taylor LF, et al. Effect of head position on vertical mandibular opening. *J Orthop Sports Phys Ther.* 1999;29(2):127-130.

Hislop HJ, Montgomery J. *Daniels and Worthingham's Muscle Testing: Techniques of Manual Examination.* 8th ed. Saunders; 2007.

Hollinshead WH. *Textbook of Anatomy.* 3rd ed. Harper & Row; 1974.

Hollis M, Yung P. *Patient Examination and Assessment for Therapists.* Blackwell Scientific Publications; 1985.

Hoppenfeld S. *Physical Examination of the Spine and Extremities.* Appleton-Century-Crofts; 1976.

Hopson MM, McPoil TG, Cornwall MW. Motion of the first metatarsophalangeal joint. Reliability and validity of four measurement techniques. *J Am Podiatr Med Assoc.* 1995;85(4):198-204.

Iddings DM, Smith LK, Spencer WA. Muscle testing: part 2. Reliability in clinical use. *Phys Ther Rev.* 1961;41:249-256.

Jepsen JR, Laursen LH, Larsen AI, et al. Manual strength testing in 14 upper limb muscles: a study of inter-rater reliability. *Acta Orthop Scand.* 2004;75:442-448.

Kapandji IA. *The Physiology of the Joints.* 5th ed. Vol. 1. Upper limb. Churchill Livingstone; 1982.

Kapandji IA. *The Physiology of the Joints.* 5th ed. Vol. 2. Lower limb. Churchill Livingstone; 1987.

Kendall FP, Kendall HO, Wadsworth GE. *Muscle Testing and Function.* 2nd ed. Williams & Wilkins; 1971.

Kendall FP, McCreary EK, Provance PG, et al. *Muscles: Testing and Function With Posture and Pain.* 5th ed. Lippincott, Williams & Wilkins; 2005.

Krusen FH, Kottke FJ, Ellwood PM. *Handbook of Physical Medicine and Rehabilitation.* 2nd ed. WB Saunders; 1971.

Lehmkuhl LD, Smith LK. *Brunnstrom's Clinical Kinesiology.* 4th ed. F.A. Davis; 1983.

Levangie P, Norkin C. *Joint Structure and Function: A Comprehensive Analysis.* 3rd ed. F.A. Davis; 2001.

Lilienfeld AM, Jacobs BA, Willis M. A study of the reproducibility of muscle testing and certain other aspects of muscle scoring. *Phys Ther Rev.* 1954;34:279-289.

Lippert LS. *Clinical Kinesiology and Anatomy.* 4th ed. F.A. Davis; 2006.

Lovett RW, Martin EG. Certain aspects of infantile paralysis with a description of a method of muscle testing. *JAMA.* 1916;66:729-733.

Lunsford BR, Perry J. The standing heel-raise test for ankle plantar flexion: criterion for normal. *Phys Ther.* 1995;75:694-698.

Magee DJ, Manske RC. *Orthopedic Physical Assessment.* 7th ed. Elsevier; 2020.

Magee DJ, Zachazewski JE, Quillen WS. *Scientific Principles of Practice in Musculoskeletal Rehabilitation.* Elsevier; 2007.

Mallon WJ, Brown H, Nunley JA. Digital ranges of motion: normal values in young adults. *J Hand Surg.* 1991;16A(5):882-887.

Moore KL, Dalley AF, Agur AMR. *Clinically Oriented Anatomy.* 8th ed. Lippincott, Williams & Wilkins; 2018.

Moore ML. The measurement of joint motion: part II—the technic of goniometry. *Phys Ther Rev.* 1949;29(6):256-264.

Mulroy SJ, Lassen KD, Chambers SH, et al. The ability of male and female clinicians to effectively test knee extension strength using manual muscle testing. *J Orthop Sports Phys Ther.* 1997;26:192-199.

Nicholas JA, Sapega A, Kraus H, et al. Factors influencing manual muscle tests in physical therapy. *J Bone Joint Surg.* 1978;60:186-190.

Norkin CC, White DJ. *Measurement of Joint Motion.* 2nd ed. F.A. Davis; 1995.

O'Sullivan SB, Schmitz TJ. *Physical Rehabilitation: Assessment and Treatment.* 3rd ed. F.A. Davis; 1994.

O'Sullivan SB, Schmitz TJ, Fulk, G. *Physical Rehabilitation.* 6th ed. F.A. Davis; 2014.

Palmer LM, Epler ME. *Clinical Assessment Procedures in Physical Therapy.* J.B. Lippincott & Co; 1990.

Palmer LM, Epler ME. *Fundamentals of Musculoskeletal Techniques.* 2nd ed. Lippincott-Raven Publishers; 1998.

Piva SR, Fitzgerald K, Irrgang, JJ, et al. Reliability of measures of impairments associated with patellofemoral pain syndrome. *BMC Musculoskelet Disord.* 2006;7:33.

Prentice WE, Voight ML. *Techniques in Musculoskeletal Rehabilitation.* McGraw-Hill; 2001.

Reese NB. *Muscle and Sensory Testing.* 4th ed. Elsevier; 2020.

Reider B. *The Orthopaedic Physical Examination.* 2nd ed. Saunders; 2005.

Reynolds PMG. Measurement of spinal mobility: a comparison of three methods. *Rheumatol Rehabil.* 1975;14:180-185.

Roaas A, Anderson GBJ. Normal range of motion of the hip, knee and ankle joints in male subjects, 30-40 years of age. *Acta Orthopaedica.* 1982;53(2):205-208.

Roach KE, Miles TP. Normal hip and knee active range of motion: the relationship to age. *Phys Ther.* 1991;71(9):656-664.

Rothstein JM. *Measurement in Physical Therapy.* Churchill Livingstone; 1985.

Rothstein JM, Roy SH, Wolf SL. *The Rehabilitation Specialist's Handbook.* 2nd ed. F.A. Davis; 1998.

Roy SH, Wolf SL, Scalzitti DA. *The Rehabilitation Specialist's Handbook.* 4th ed. F.A. Davis; 2013.

Salter N. Methods of measurement of muscle and joint function. *J Bone Joint Surg Br.* 1955;34:474.

Sapega AA. Muscle performance evaluation in orthopedic practice. *J Bone Joint Surg.* 1990;72:1562-1574.

Schenker AW. Goniometry—an improved method of joint measurement. *N Y State J Med.* 1956;56(4):539-545.

Schwartz S, Cohen ME, Herbison GJ, et al. Relationship between two measures of upper extremity strength: manual muscle test compared to hand-held myometry. *Arch Phys Med Rehabil.* 1992;73:1063-1068.

Sieg KW, Adams SP. *Illustrated Essentials of Musculoskeletal Anatomy.* 4th ed. Megabooks; 2002.

Smidt GC, Rogers MW. Factors contributing to the regulation and clinical assessment of muscle strength. *Phys Ther.* 1982;62:1283-1289.

Smith LK, Weiss EL, Lehmkuhl DL. *Brunnstrom's Clinical Kinesiology.* 5th ed. F.A. Davis; 1996.

Van Ost L. *Cram Session in Goniometry: A Handbook for Student and Clinicians.* SLACK Incorporated; 2010.

Van Ost L. *Goniometry.* SLACK Incorporated; 1999.

Wadsworth CT, Krishnan R, Sear R, et al. Intrarater reliability of manual muscle testing and hand-held dynamic muscle testing. *Phys Ther.* 1987;67:1342-1347.

Walker N, Bohannon RW, Cameron D. Discriminant validity of temporomandibular joint range of motion measurements obtained with a ruler. *J Orthop Sports Phys Ther.* 2000;30(8):484-492.

Watkins MA, Riddle DL, Lamb RL, et al. Reliability of goniometric measurements and visual estimates of knee range of motion obtained in a clinical setting. *Phys Ther.* 1991;71(2):90-97.

West CC. Measurement of joint motion. *Arch Phys Med Rehabil.* 1945;26:414.

Williams M. Manual muscle testing, development and current use. *Phys Ther Rev.* 1956;36:797-805.

Williams M, Stutzman L. Strength variation through the range of motion. *Phys Ther Rev.* 1959;39:145-152.

Wintz MM. Variations in current manual muscle testing. *Phys Ther Rev.* 1959;39:466-475.

Youdas JW, Carey JR, Garrett TR. Reliability of measurements of cervical spine range of motion—comparison of three methods. *Phys Ther.* 1991;71(2):98-104.

Youdas JW, Garrett TR, Suman VJ, et al. Normal range of motion of the cervical spine: an initial goniometric study. *Phys Ther.* 1992;72(11):770-780.

Zimny N, Kirk C. A comparison of methods of manual muscle testing. *Clin Manag Phys Ther.* 1987;7(2):6-11.

# Index

Printed in the United States
by Baker & Taylor Publisher Services